Feed Your Baby & Toddler Right

Early eating and drinking skills encourage the best development

Diane Bahr, MS, CCC-SLP

author of *Nobody Ever Told Me (or My Mother) That!*

Feed Your Baby & Toddler Right is a partial update/edition of the book *Nobody Ever Told Me (or My Mother) That! Everything from Bottles and Breathing to Healthy Speech Development.*

All marketing and publishing rights guaranteed to and reserved by:

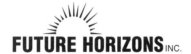

FUTURE HORIZONS INC.

721 W Abram St, Arlington, TX 76013

800-489-0727 (toll free)

817-277-0727 (local)

817-277-2270 (fax)

E-mail: *info@fhautism.com*

www.fhautism.com

ISBN: 9781941765678

Dedication

This book is dedicated to all of the wonderful children, families, and professionals with whom I have had the pleasure to work. I wish to particularly thank my husband Joe and my daughter Kim, who provide me with the ongoing support and care I need to continue to do the work I enjoy.

Advance Praise for
Feed Your Baby & Toddler Right

Diane has done it again! Her new book, *Feed Your Baby & Toddler Right*, is a valuable tool for any parent or professional. She outlines first-years' development details and characteristics like no other resource. I love the ages and stages check sheets and write-in charts. She tells me exactly what my child needs to be doing and when—very helpful. Most importantly, she shares practical solutions not only on how to effectively breastfeed and/or bottle-feed, but how to transition into spoon-feeding, cup-drinking, straw-drinking, chewing, and swallowing. A highly recommended resource!

> — **Char Boshart, MA, CCC-SLP**
> **Speech-Language Pathologist, Author, Lecturer**
> **Ellijay, Georgia, USA**

Diane's latest book is extremely helpful, educational, and easy to understand. She highlights so many issues other books don't even address. We started working with her a year ago with our son who had speech delays. It was amazing to learn that his delays were attributed to something as simple as a tongue-tie or sucking pads. We wish we had been aware of these issues and easy steps to take earlier in his development. This book is a great resource for parents to ensure the best development of their child. We really love the developmental checklists to help a parent understand typical milestones, potential pitfalls, and recommended solutions. Children don't come with instruction books, but this book provides great insight into oral development. We are so grateful for Diane's expertise and highly recommend this book to every parent.

> — **Samantha and Steve Broderick**
> **Parents**
> **Las Vegas, Nevada, USA**

This book is an excellent and useful tool with appropriate guidelines for all families with infants and toddlers. The foundation for optimal orofacial growth and development begins with early eating and drinking skills. Diane Bahr, MS, CCC-SLP has a vast array of experience and expertise in this area which will be useful for many healthcare professionals as well.

> — **Marge Foran, RDH, COM**
> **Dental Professional, Certified Orofacial Myologist**
> **Montana, USA**

Diane Bahr's expertise helps parents appreciate the complex, yet amazing capabilities of the babies and children they are responsible for properly feeding. I'm incredibly thankful for Diane's commitment to review and summarize thousands of pages of current research into simple, easy-to-understand checklists. Her book is packed with numerous tools and invaluable knowledge related to feeding and mouth development. This book is a treasure for any parent or child-development professional.

> — **Julia Franklin, MS, CCC-SLP**
> **Speech-Language Pathologist**
> **Charlotte, North Carolina, USA**

As a parent, clinician, lecturer, and advocate for understanding appropriate feeding skills and intervention, I value all the work Diane has continued to share with the public. Her simple explanations of complex topics help both parents and professionals better understand the steps of intervention. Her expertise continues to guide the field of feeding, and her willingness to share her knowledge is steadfast. Each chapter of her new book, *Feed Your Baby & Toddler Right*, provides specific information regarding development and practical introduction of foods and liquids. I look forward to sharing her information with parents and medical professionals for many years to come.

> — **Kristie Gatto, MA, CCC-SLP, COM**
> **Speech-Language Pathologist, Certified**
> **Orofacial Myologist, Author, Lecturer**
> **President of the International Association of**
> **Orofacial Myology**
> **Texas, USA**

Diane Bahr's *Feed Your Baby & Toddler Right* is a concise and practical book for parents and professionals alike. The format provides an overview of the developmental feeding stages from babyhood to toddler-age children. Her feeding competencies designed in a checklist format provide parents, caregivers, and professionals an easy reference from which to work. Access to sources for services and tools recommended are easily identifiable in the text. Diane's knowledge and experience have made possible this comprehensive, yet simple and accessible book for everyone. Her reference bibliography gives the reader a glimpse of her thoroughness and dedication in the writing of this book.

> — **Rosalba D. Gutierrez, MS, IBCLC**
> **International Board-Certified Lactation**
> **Consultant**
> **Texas, USA**

Diane's book demonstrates the depth and specialism of her work. She covers each key topic in great detail and in a way that makes this book required reading for both parents and professionals. Of particular use are the key developmental checklists and the links to specialists and additional resources/tools. It has been my great pleasure to work with Diane for a number of years. Her specialist knowledge, highly effective problem-solving approach, and generous spirit are making a big difference for a member of my family.

> — **Dr. Margaret Hobson, MEd, PhD**
> **Education Consultant**
> **United Kingdom**

This information about feeding in Diane's book *Feed Your Baby & Toddler Right* is invaluable, both for my typically developing child and my child with special needs. I wish I would have had these concise guidelines and checklists from the beginning. Feeding would have been much less overwhelming!

> — **Kate Jacobs**
> **Parent**
> **Las Vegas, Nevada, USA**

How we feed our babies and transition them to solids is crucial to their development. Diane's newest book is definitive, evidence-based, and easy to follow. Parents have a lot to navigate these days, especially with social media, so this book by one of our leading experts in the field of pediatric feeding is a must-have!

— Nina Ayd Johanson, MS, MA, CCC-SLP; CEIM; CHHP
Speech-Language Pathologist, Pediatric Feeding Specialist,
Certified Infant Massage Instructor, Lecturer
Baltimore, Maryland, USA

Diane Bahr communicates the vital topic of infant and toddler nourishment with thoroughness and sensitive consideration of the reader. Parents will find the language easy to follow and the content encouraging, thus providing a sense of empowerment—something that is critical in any aspect of parenting. Diane's books have also been highly regarded among many healthcare professionals, and her approach toward best functional outcomes is outstanding. I will definitely share her book with my patients.

— Dr. Marjan Jones
Integrative Dentist, Lecturer
Australia

Diane has written a clear, easy-to-understand guide of oral sensory-motor skill development for successful feeding. This book should be in the library of every parent who desires to approach overall healthcare in a preventative manner. So many of our mouth development, feeding, and dental (malocclusions) problems could be prevented or minimized by early and appropriate feeding. I will be purchasing one for my son, his wife, and my first grandchild.

— Phyllis J. Magelky, MS, CCC-SLP, COM
Speech-Language Pathologist, Certified Orofacial Myologist
Fargo, North Dakota, USA

I loved reading Diane Bahr's new book, and parents will love having this book on hand as their baby develops. Not only will parents learn the how, what, and when of feeding skills, they will also understand why it is so very important to establish good feeding skills early and how that relates to healthy airway development. Parents will love the blow-by-blow explanations of what babies can do, when to expect it, and how to help them do it with lots of practical tips. This book is not just for parents. Professionals who work with babies and young children will appreciate the deep, clinical, detail-derived information from Di's extensive clinical experience. It may also serve as a wonderful teaching tool for healthcare practitioners who are learning how to work "in the mouths of babes." Congratulations, Di, very well done.

— Sharon Moore, CPSP
Speech Pathologist, Lecturer
Author of Sleep Wrecked Kids
Australia

The book *Feed Your Baby & Toddler Right* contains unique health information that parents, the public, and healthcare professionals need to know. It furthers the understanding of what Dr. Charles H. Mayo said in 1934 about the value of oral health in disease prevention. Even today, the Mayo Clinic says overall health reflects oral health. Diane Bahr, an oral and overall health pioneer, continues the quest for better health at the earliest treatable age.

— Dr. David C. Page, Sr.
Functional Jaw Orthopedist, Integrative Dentist, Lecturer
Author of Your Jaws - Your Life
Baltimore, MD, USA

As a bodyworker and TummyTime! Method professional specializing in treating tongue-tied babies, I found Diane's book *Feed Your Baby & Toddler Right* extremely useful. Along with her first book, *Nobody Ever Told Me (or My Mother) That!*, I have gained a strong foundation in oral development and function which has helped me to identify when babies should be referred for appropriate services such as speech or occupational therapy. Diane's new book is a profound multidisciplinary resource that covers everything from reflex integration to the progression of feeding; from motor planning for breastfeeding vs. bottle feeding to trouble-shooting either option; and from tongue-tie to intentional tummy time. Diane's books continue to be ongoing resources for me professionally and personally as a mother of two tongue-tied children. I have worked extensively with Di, and so it really is a pleasure and an honor to review her material. Her expertise has allowed me to become a powerful, educated advocate for tongue-tied babies. I highly recommend *Feed Your Baby & Toddler Right* for all parents and professionals working in the field of pediatrics.

> — **Sara Riley, LMT**
> **Licensed Massage Therapist, TummyTime! Method Professional/**
> **Teaching Assistant**
> **Dartmouth, Massachusetts, USA**

Diane Bahr's new book, *Feed Your Baby & Toddler Right*, is an invaluable resource in outlining the benefits of proper child feeding. As a product of her conscientious research, Diane has staked her position as a trusted, knowledgeable voice in the vanguard of pediatric oral sensory-motor assessment and treatment. Her desire to cultivate a generation of healthy children free of feeding, speech, and mouth development pathologies materializes through offering parents and clinicians alike a pragmatic educational set of the best possible practices.

> — **Sanda Valcu-Pinkerton, RDHAP, OMT**
> **Dental and Orofacial Myofunctional Professional, Lecturer**
> **The Breathe Institute**
> **Los Angeles, California, USA**

Diane Bahr has done truly outstanding work in gathering the evidence-based literature with perspectives of various thought-leaders into an actionable checklist for parents to learn how the simple acts of eating and drinking can impact a child's long-term orofacial health and airway development. This book is a comprehensive resource on feeding, speech, oral sensory-motor skills, and functional development, written in a style that is accessible by parents and professionals alike. I implore mothers, fathers, and educational/clinical leaders to congratulate Diane for her steadfast dedication to child development and oral health. I am truly honored to collaborate with and learn from such a dedicated visionary!

> — **Dr. Soroush Zaghi, MD, ENT**
> **Sleep Surgeon, Airway Centric Otolaryngologist, Lecturer**
> **The Breathe Institute**
> **Los Angeles, California, USA**

Reader's Note

This book reflects the ideas and opinions of the author. Its purpose is to give the reader helpful information on the topics covered in the book. It is not meant to provide health, medical, or professional consultation. The reader is advised to consult appropriate health, medical, and other professionals for these processes. The author and publisher do not take responsibility for any personal or other risk, loss, or liability incurred as a direct or indirect consequence of application or use of information found in this book.

Acknowledgements

I would like to acknowledge the many extraordinary people who assisted me in the completion of this book. If I have forgotten anyone, I sincerely apologize.

To those who read, reviewed, and made suggestions for appropriate sections of the book:

Char Boshart, Speech-Language Pathologist, Author, Lecturer

Kelley Carter, Speech-Language Pathologist, Certified Orofacial Myologist

Marge Foran, Dental Professional, Certified Orofacial Myologist

Dee Dee Franke, International Board-Certified Lactation Consultant

Julia Franklin, Speech-Language Pathologist

Kristie Gatto, Speech-Language Pathologist, Certified Orofacial Myologist, Author, Lecturer

Catherine Watson Genna, International Board-Certified Lactation Consultant, Author, Lecturer

Rosabla Gutierrez, International Board-Certified Lactation Consultant

Kenda Hammer, Educator

David Hammer, Speech-Language Pathologist, Lecturer

Nina Ayd Johanson, Speech-Language Pathologist, Certified Infant Massage Instructor, Lecturer

Marjan Jones, Integrative Dentist, Lecturer

Sandra Kahn, Integrative Othodontist, Lecturer

Lawrence A. Kotlow, Pediatric Dentist, Author, Lecturer

Phyllis Magelky, Speech-Language Pathologist, Certified Orofacial Myologist

David C. Page, Sr., Functional Jaw Orthopedist, Integrative Dentist, Author, Lecturer

Barry Raphael, Integrative Orthodontist, Lecturer

Autumn Wake, International Board-Certified Lactation Consultant

Simon Wong, Integrative Dentist, Lecturer

Soroush Zaghi, Airway Centric Otolaryngologist, Sleep Surgeon, Lecturer

To those who provided advance praise for the book:

Char Boshart, Speech-Language Pathologist, Author, Lecturer

Samantha and Steve Broderick, Parents

Marge Foran, Dental Professional, Certified Orofacial Myologist

Julia Franklin, Speech-Language Pathologist

Kristie Gatto, Speech-Language Pathologist, Certified Orofacial Myologist, Author, Lecturer

Rosabla Gutierrez, International Board-Certified Lactation Consultant

Margaret Hobson, Education Consultant

Kate Jacobs, Parent

Nina Ayd Johanson, Speech-Language Pathologist, Certified Infant Massage Instructor, Lecturer

Marjan Jones, Integrative Dentist, Lecturer

Phyllis Magelky, Speech-Language Pathologist, Certified Orofacial Myologist

Sharon Moore, Speech Pathologist, Author, Lecturer

David C. Page, Sr., Functional Jaw Orthopedist, Integrative Dentist, Author, Lecturer

Sara Riley, Licensed Massage Therapist, Tummy Time! Method Professional/Teaching Assistant

Sanda Valcu-Pinkerton, Dental and Orofacial Myofunctional Professional

Soroush Zaghi, Airway Centric Otolaryngologist, Sleep Surgeon, Lecturer

To those who provided drawings, photos, and images with permission for the book:

Kimberly DeFriez, Parent, Speech-Language Pathologist, Information Technology Specialist

Tarik DeFriez, Parent, Information Technology Specialist

Alison Deleon, Parent

Eastland Press

Cristiane Fotia, Parent

Anthony Fotia, Sr., Parent, Artist

Bobak (Bobby) Ghaheri, Airway Centric Otolaryngologist

Lawrence (Larry) A. Kotlow, Pediatric Dentist, Author, Lecturer

Rebecca Lowsky of ARK Therapeutic

Suzanne Evans Morris, Speech-Language Pathologist, Feeding Specialist, Author, Lecturer

David C. Page, Sr., Functional Jaw Orthopedist, Integrative Dentist, Author, Lecturer

To the wonderful folks at Future Horizons who made this book possible. Thank you, Jennifer, Lyn, Rose, Morgan, and the many others who took part in this process.

Contents

Contents

Foreword

When we sat down to write *Raising a Healthy, Happy Eater*, we both realized parents needed a solid understanding of how their child would progress through various stages of development and, just as importantly, how that would affect their feeding experience. We are Melanie (Coach Mel), a childhood feeding specialist, and Nimali (Doctor Yum), a pediatrician focused on teaching healthy eating.

We teamed up to help parents set their kids on the path to adventurous eating from birth or to gently guide their older kids back on track if they were having difficulties. As we typed away, shaping the roadmap that would become our book, the one reference we had near our respective laptops was Diane Bahr's book *Nobody Ever Told Me (or My Mother) That! Everything from Bottles and Breathing to Healthy Speech Development*. For Coach Mel, it's her bible for understanding mouth development, and it's a valuable resource on the shelves in Doctor Yum's pediatric office.

As professionals who take care of children every day, we embrace the importance of early development in a child's journey to becoming a great eater. We were fortunate to receive literature-based information in our training and then apply it in practice every day when assessing and treating children.

Unfortunately, parents may not receive that same information about development despite the fact they are also assessing and interacting with their children every day. Parents want information—and Diane's new book, *Feed Your Baby & Toddler Right*, is the most extensive, research-backed source on bookshelves today. Moms and Dads will find crucial developmental checklists, expert information on breastfeeding and bottle-feeding, and how to problem solve if something doesn't seem right before advancing to solid foods.

Whether parents decide to breastfeed or bottle-feed, understanding the development of the mouth can help their babies have a successful feeding experience from day one. Armed with a good reference like *Feed Your Baby & Toddler Right*, parents can identify issues and enact solutions before more serious problems develop.

As children progress with their feeding skills, it's important for parents to understand how development shapes skills for spoon-feeding, open cup-drinking, drinking from a straw, as well as chewing and swallowing solid foods. As with many areas of child development, identifying problems early and timely intervention are key. Oral sensory-motor skills and feeding are no exception. Feeding is an important part of the human experience, which we share many times a day as a family. Therefore, raising a child to enjoy healthy food at mealtimes makes life at home more peaceful, less stressful, and more memorable. When kids enjoy a variety of healthy foods, it sets them on a path for a healthy body and mind for life.

The book *Feed Your Baby & Toddler Right* brings the professional eye of Diane Bahr into every household. Diane guides parents through mouth development, ensuring their baby or toddler grows and develops in the best way possible—with healthy feeding development from the very start. We are so pleased to share Diane's latest resource with you and wish you and your family the happiest of mealtimes.

> — **Doctor Yum and Coach Mel**
> Co-authors of *Raising a Healthy, Happy Eater: A Stage-by-Stage Guide to Setting Your Child on the Path to Adventurous Eating*

Introduction

As a feeding and speech therapist for almost forty years, I've seen many children with health and development concerns directly related to problems with feeding and other early mouth experiences. These include tongue, lip, and buccal ties, sinus and ear problems, allergies and sensitivities, asthma, gastroesophageal reflux, sleep-disordered breathing, picky and selective eating leading to nutritional problems, late feeding and mouth development, as well as orthodontic issues. Many of these problems could be avoided or reduced if parents and professionals had more information and training in the specifics of feeding, mouth, and airway development.

This book contains the best research I could find. In the book, I tell you the secrets many feeding professionals have learned over the years, which the typical parent may never hear and a child's pediatrician may not know. While there are many books on breastfeeding, childhood nutrition, and child development, this book details the mechanics of feeding and mouth development which hopefully assists good airway development. Good feeding techniques and appropriate mouth activities are essential for a child's overall health, well-being, and development.

Today, parents often do not have the role models of extended families living nearby to demonstrate techniques used successfully by previous generations. This information is not innate in our modern world, and feeding can become a tedious pattern of trial and error for parents and their children if they don't have help.

Just ask some parents, particularly moms:

1. Why did you choose bottle-feeding over breastfeeding despite wanting to breastfeed?

2. How many bottles did you try before finding one that worked?

3. How did you learn about introducing foods and liquids at appropriate ages and times?

4. How many of you have children who are picky or selective eaters?

There are horror stories about children who refuse to eat an appropriate variety of foods necessary for basic nutrition. Many of these struggles began with incorrect and/or unsuccessful early feeding techniques. Speech-language pathologists are also seeing many children with late-developing speech. These are often the same children who have feeding problems.

The ideas presented in this book help parents and professionals solve these problems easily and naturally. Giving parents and professionals appropriate tools to feed babies and toddlers decrease parent anxiety and frustration. It also increases positive interactions between parents and their children. In his book *The Happiest Baby on the Block*, Dr. Harvey Karp says parents who succeed in feeding and calming their babies "feel proud, confident, and on top of the world!"[1]

By using the simple, appropriate techniques presented in this book, you will help your child develop:

1. Good mouth and airway structures that support overall health.

2. Appropriate eating and drinking skills used throughout life.

Just follow the simple, healthy guidelines in the book as you go through your everyday activities with your child. They will make your life easier and eliminate guesswork. This is a guilt-free, pressure-free, success-oriented approach, so you can have fun and enjoy watching your child develop these amazing skills.

Important note for parents: If you have difficulty applying the information found in this book, seek out a feeding or other appropriate professional. If you become overwhelmed by the amount of information in the book, look up one piece of information at a time as it applies to you and your baby or toddler.

Important note for professionals: This book is meant to be used with parents, so please use it as needed to guide the parents with whom you work. Additionally, please feel free to use this book as a curriculum in teaching parent and professional groups. It takes a village to help our modern world *get back on track* with appropriate feeding and mouth development.

1

Crucial Developmental Checklists

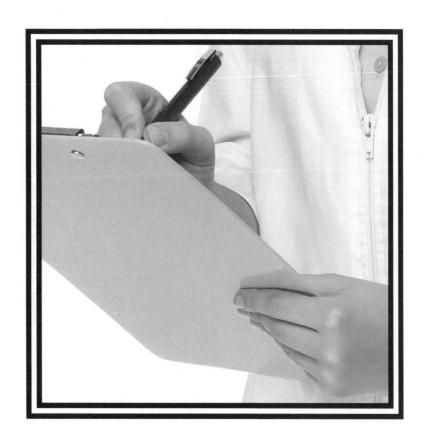

What This Book Can Do for You

Parents often receive little instruction on how to feed their children, yet good feeding, eating, and drinking skills encourage the best possible mouth development. You are going to feed your child, so why not use appropriate feeding techniques to support your child's mouth development from birth?

Most of our eating and drinking skills develop in the first 2 years of life. Your child's feeding skills will change rapidly, particularly in the first year. However, many parents don't know the significance of these rapid changes. You can help with the process by using appropriate feeding methods.

Feeding is like dancing. You and your child are partners in this dance. The best feeding method for you and your child may be somewhat different from what others do. As in ballroom dancing, many of the steps are similar, but you will use specific feeding variations to suit you and your child.

This book contains important guidelines to help you and your child learn the *feeding dance* easily and successfully. It also addresses problems you may encounter in feeding. Some information is repeated in the book for your convenience.

The Importance of Developmental Checklists

We begin with some crucial developmental checklists, so you can discover how your infant or toddler is doing. The checklists are approximate and not absolute. Every baby and toddler has his or her own unique developmental sequence.

If your child is not on track according to the checklists, other sections in the book provide the specific information you need. There are sections on breastfeeding, bottle-feeding, spoon-feeding, cup- and straw-drinking, finger-feeding, taking bites of food, chewing, picky or selective eating, and so on.

Checklists are a good place to begin your journey as they reflect *typical development* recorded in the literature. You will see where your baby is on track in development. You will also see skills you may want to help him or her develop. The following developmental checklists are found in this chapter of the book:

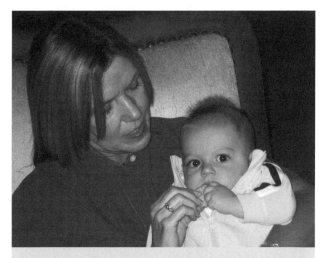

Photo 1.1: *Anthony (age 6 months) eats his first arrowroot baby cookie while holding it with Diane. They are partners in the feeding dance.*

• Feeding and Related Development Checklist: Birth to 24 Months

- Food and Liquid Introduction Checklist: Birth to 24 Months

- Intentional, Supervised Tummy/Belly Time to Creeping/Crawling Checklist:

  A Likely Fundamental Missing Developmental Link (Birth to 7 Months)

- Mouth and Hand-Mouth Reflex or Response Checklists

Feeding and Related Development Checklist: Birth-24 Months [2 3 4 5 6 7 8 9 10 11 12 13 14 15 16 17 18 19]

This checklist is a guide to help you gauge if your child is *on track* in feeding development. The details presented in these lists are available to therapists, but most parents and pediatricians don't have the benefit of this literature-based, criterion-referenced information. Many resources were used to create these checklists. A special thank-you goes to Suzanne Evans Morris, who supplied the only known longitudinal study on typical feeding development.[20] She and Marsha Dunn Klein wrote *Pre-Feeding Skills: A Comprehensive Resource for Mealtime Development (2nd ed.)*, which continues to be a primary reference for feeding specialists and was a vital resource for this book.[21]

If you have questions concerning your child's feeding development, please discuss these with your child's pediatrician and appropriate other professionals as needed.

Place a check mark next to the characteristics you see in your baby at birth.

BIRTH: A FULL-TERM BABY (40 WEEKS GESTATION)	CHECK MARK
Mouth and throat structures are close together as a protective mechanism during feeding.	☐
Has functional maturity in sucking, swallowing, and breathing coordination.	☐
Breastfeeds (best feeding method for a baby's health and development); laid-back position seems most natural.	☐
Bottle-feeds (medical feeding method); paced (baby-led) bottle-feeding with baby held upright at a 45+ degree angle to the horizon (not lying down) is recommended if bottle-feeding.	☐
Tongue cups breast or bottle nipple during sucking.	☐
Gums may enlarge to assist with the latch (likely related to increased blood supply in gums).	☐

BIRTH: A FULL-TERM BABY (40 WEEKS GESTATION) continued	CHECK MARK
Lips latch properly on breast or bottle (somewhat different for breastfeeding than bottle-feeding).	☐
Nutritive suck is approximately 1 per second; non-nutritive suckle is approximately 2 per second.	☐
May have some liquid loss from mouth.	☐
Has a full set of sucking or fat pads in cheeks for side-mouth stability.	☐
Participates in generalized mouthing—mouths hands and fingers near front of mouth.	☐
Has easy nose-breathing.	☐
Mouth is closed during sleep and when mouth is inactive (not feeding, mouthing hands, or making vocal sounds).	☐
Tongue rests in the roof of the mouth to help maintain the broad palate shape (pacifier or bottle nipples cannot do this, but proper breastfeeding assists in maintaining the palate's shape).	☐
Free of tethered oral tissues, such as tongue tie (important to check at birth).	☐
Baby has a good amount of intentional, supervised tummy or belly time, as well as other body positions to ensure adequate and on-time development of sensory-motor skills.	☐
Typical body, mouth, and hand-mouth reflexes are present (pediatrician can check).	☐

At birth, your baby's mouth and throat structures are close together to protect him or her from choking when feeding. Feeding readiness is based on the coordination of sucking, swallowing, and breathing. If feeding well, your baby's tongue will cup the breast or bottle nipple (not hump or bunch). Her gums may enlarge to assist with the latch. This is likely related to increased blood supply to the gums. Her lips will latch on the bottle nipple or breast. She will suck approximately 1 time per second (nutritive suck) but may lose some liquid from her mouth when feeding. If she suckles faster, such as 2 times per second, she may not be getting milk (non-nutritive suckle).

Full-term, typically developing babies (40 weeks gestation) usually have the innate ability to breastfeed (unless there is a tongue tie or other problem at birth). In my opinion, babies should be checked for reflexes, sucking pads, nose-breathing, and tethered oral tissues (particularly tongue ties) at birth.

When babies are placed on the mom's abdomen right after birth, they usually crawl to the breast and begin feeding.[22][23][24] The umbilical cord may be attached and pulsing for a period of time after birth.[25] Breastfeeding is biologically normal, and the best way to feed a baby for the most ideal health and development. The laid-back breastfeeding position seems to be the most natural. If you wish to breastfeed, work with an International Board-Certified Lactation Consultant (IBCLC) and feeding specialist if needed.

Babies who are close to term (37 to 39 weeks) or premature can also learn to breastfeed with appropriate help. Sucking or fat pads develop in a baby's cheeks toward the end of a full-term pregnancy. These provide the side-stability in the mouth needed particularly for breastfeeding. Many babies who are close to term do not have adequate sucking pads. Babies born prematurely usually do not have sucking pads. Accommodations for this problem, such as carefully applied cheek support, are covered in this book.

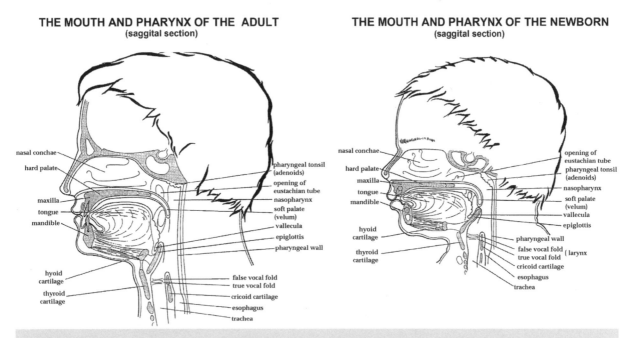

THE MOUTH AND PHARYNX OF THE ADULT
(saggital section)

THE MOUTH AND PHARYNX OF THE NEWBORN
(saggital section)

Figure 1.1: *There are significant structural differences between a full-term newborn (40 weeks gestation) and the adult mouth and throat. The newborn is ready for breastfeeding and medical bottle-feeding (if and when needed). Drawings developed by Artist Betsy True for Suzanne Evans Morris who granted permission for their use.*

Unfortunately, many families are encouraged to bottle-feed their babies, particularly if the baby does not immediately breastfeed at birth. Bottle-feeding is an unnatural, medical way of feeding a baby. It's a very different process from breastfeeding. If you are bottle-feeding, be sure your baby's ear is above her mouth as you hold her body upright at a 45+ degree angle to the horizon (not lying down). This will help keep liquid from going into her Eustachian tubes and middle ears, which may cause ear problems. Paced (baby-led) bottle-feeding is recommended. Please read the breastfeeding and bottle-feeding sections in this book.

Your baby will mouth her hands and fingers near the front of her mouth (generalized mouthing). When your baby is not feeding, sucking on fingers and/or hands, or making vocal sounds, her mouth should be closed. Then her tongue can rest in the roof of her mouth to help maintain a typical broad palate shape. She will be nose-breathing, which is crucial for good health. Mouth-breathing, on the other hand, is extremely unhealthy.[26][27][28][29][30] Proper breastfeeding also assists in maintaining the palate's shape.

Additionally, your baby's mouth should be free of tethered oral tissues, such as tongue tie. If your baby's tongue is tied, it cannot rest in the roof of the mouth to help maintain the palate's broad shape. This often results in high and narrow mouth roof, which makes the nasal area small and impacts healthy nasal breathing.

Your baby also needs a good amount of supervised, intentional tummy or belly time, as well as other body positions, to ensure adequate and on-time development of sensory-motor skills. The development of postural control in the body is the foundation for movement. It leads to rolling, sitting, and the refined skills your child will eventually develop in the mouth, eyes, and hands (eating, drinking, babbling, vision use, self-feeding, etc.).

At birth, your baby will have full-body reflexes, in addition to 3 hand-mouth reflexes and 7 mouth (or oral) reflexes. Your child's pediatrician or other appropriate professionals can check these. All of the reflexes are important for the development of postural (or body) control and feeding.

The 3 hand-mouth reflexes are the *palmomental*, *Babkin*, and *grasp*. These reflexes help your baby's hands and mouth work together during feeding. The 7 mouth (or oral) reflexes are *rooting*, *suckling*, *tongue extrusion*, *swallowing*, *phasic bite*, *transverse tongue*, and *gag*. These reflexes assist with feeding. At birth, your baby's gag response will be found on the back ¾ of her tongue to protect her from ingesting items too large to swallow. You have a chart on the 7 mouth reflexes and 3 hand-mouth reflexes for your reference near the end of this chapter.

Place a check mark next to the characteristics you see in your baby at 1 month of age.

1 MONTH	CHECK MARK
Control of rooting reflex developing (rooting leads to sucking).	☐
Easily locates nipple with mouth.	☐
Sucks thin liquid from the bottle or breast sequencing 2 or more sucks.	☐
May still lose some liquid from the mouth.	☐
Participates in generalized mouthing—mouths hands and fingers near front of mouth.	☐
Baby's mouth, nose, and throat areas are growing and changing.	☐
Baby has easy nose-breathing.	☐
Mouth is closed during sleep and when mouth is inactive (not feeding, mouthing hands, or making vocal sounds).	☐
Tongue rests in the roof of the mouth to help maintain the broad palate shape (pacifier or bottle nipple cannot do this, but proper breastfeeding can).	☐
Baby is free of tethered oral tissues, such as tongue tie.	☐
Baby has a good amount of intentional, supervised tummy or belly time as well as other body positions to ensure adequate and on-time development of sensory-motor skills.	☐
Baby can imitate some mouth movement (open mouth, tongue out) and can match the pitch and duration of your voice.[31]	☐

By 1 month of age, your baby can locate the breast or bottle nipple easily with his or her mouth. The rooting reflex is coming under control. You will see the rooting reflex more often in breastfed than bottle-fed babies unless paced (baby-led) bottle-feeding is used. Breastfed babies use the rooting reflex to find the mother's nipple. Bottle-fed babies often have the nipple placed into their mouths and don't really use the reflex unless the parent is using suggested and preferred paced (baby-led) bottle-feeding. Your baby can now suck breast milk or formula sequencing 2 (or usually more) sucks at a time with good suck-swallow-breathe coordination but may still lose some liquid from the mouth.

Your baby's mouth, nose, and throat areas continue to grow and change. He will mouth his hands and fingers near front of the mouth (generalized mouthing). He should have easy nose-breathing, and his mouth should be closed during sleep and when his mouth is inactive (not feeding, mouthing hands, or making vocal sounds). His tongue should rest in the roof of his mouth to help maintain the broad palate shape. A pacifier or bottle nipple cannot do this, but proper breastfeeding can help keep the palate shape. His mouth should also be free of tethered oral tissues, such as tongue tie.

Additionally, your baby requires a good amount of intentional, supervised tummy or belly time, as well as other body positions, to ensure adequate and on-time development of sensory-motor skills. This creates the foundation for the postural control required for feeding and ultimately speaking. Your baby can imitate some mouth movement (open mouth, tongue out) and can match the pitch and duration of your voice. These are likely the *mirror neurons* at work, which allow your baby to mirror what you do.

Place a check mark next to the characteristics you see in your baby at 2 to 3 months of age.

2 TO 3 MONTHS	CHECK MARK
Control of suckling reflex developing (non-nutritive, front-back tongue movement, approximately 2 per second).	☐
The mouth is beginning to change shape, and the tongue is beginning to move with increasing purpose within the mouth.	☐
Longer sucking without a pause on the bottle or breast.	☐
Brings hands together (may also be seen from birth).	☐
Participates in generalized mouthing: brings hands to front of mouth when on belly (around 2 months) and when on back (around 3 months).	☐
Baby's mouth, nose, and throat areas are growing and changing.	☐

2 TO 3 MONTHS continued	CHECK MARK
Baby has easy nose-breathing.	☐
Mouth is closed during sleep and when mouth is inactive (not feeding, mouthing hands, or making vocal sounds).	☐
Tongue rests in the roof of the mouth to help maintain the broad palate shape (pacifier or bottle nipples cannot do this, but proper breastfeeding can help keep the broad palate shape).	☐
Baby is free of tethered oral tissues, such as tongue tie.	☐
Baby has a good amount of intentional, supervised tummy or belly time as well as other body positions to ensure adequate and on-time development of sensory-motor skills.	☐
Baby follows parent's or care provider's movement with his or her eyes and vocalizes in response to speech.	☐

By 2 to 3 months of age, your baby is developing control of the suckling reflex. He or she will suck for longer periods of time without pausing. The mouth is beginning to change shape, and the tongue is beginning to move with increasing purpose within the mouth. You will also see your baby bring her hands together when feeding. She may rest them on the breast or bottle. Around 2 months of age, your baby will bring her hands to her mouth when she is on her belly, and around 3 months of age, she will bring her hands to her mouth when she is on her back. This process is called generalized

Photo 1.2: *Nose-breathing is essential for your child's overall health, feeding, mouth, and airway development at every age.*

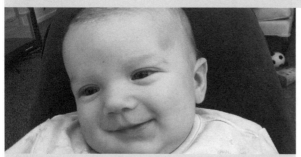

Grayson (2.5 months) is nose-breathing with lips nicely closed.

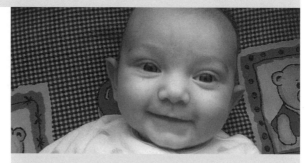

Rylee (3 months) has good nose-breathing, as well as a nice broad eye area and straight lip line indicating good upper airway and jaw development.

mouthing because your baby is mouthing or sucking on her hands at the front of her mouth. Your baby also did this in utero.

Babies with difficulty breastfeeding or bottle-feeding often improve significantly by 6 to 8 weeks of age as their suck-swallow-breathe coordination increases. You may need to work with your International Board-Certified Lactation Consultant and/or a feeding therapist to arrive at this point. Feeding therapists are usually speech-language pathologists or occupational therapists who specialize in feeding.

Your baby's mouth, nose, and throat areas continue to grow and change. She should have easy nose-breathing, and her mouth should be closed during sleep and when her mouth is inactive (not feeding, mouthing hands, or making vocal sounds). Her tongue should rest in the roof of the mouth to help maintain the palate shape. A pacifier or bottle nipple cannot do this, but proper breastfeeding can help keep the broad palate shape. Her mouth should be free of tethered oral tissues, such as tongue tie.

Additionally, your baby requires a good amount of intentional, supervised tummy or belly time as well as other body positions to ensure adequate and on-time development of sensory-motor skills. Good postural control is the foundation on which refined motor skills like feeding and ultimately speaking are developed. Your baby may follow your movements with her eyes and vocalize. This, again, may be her mirror neurons in her brain at work. Mirror neurons are those which allow your baby to copy what you do.

Place a check mark next to the characteristics you see in your baby at 3 to 6 months of age.

3 TO 6 MONTHS	CHECK MARK
DEVELOPMENT	
Tongue extrusion and Babkin reflexes seems to fade between 3 and 4 months.	☐
Rooting reflex seems to be disappearing; baby locates the breast nipple frequently without use of rooting reflex between 3 and 6 months.	☐
Third lips disappear between 3 and 6 months—third lips are a slight swelling of the gum area likely related to increased blood supply.	☐
Gag reflex comes under control with appropriate mouthing and feeding experiences between 4 and 6 months.	☐

3 TO 6 MONTHS continued	CHECK MARK
Control develops over phasic bite reflex between 5 and 9 months as baby gets ready to take bites of and chew foods.	☐
Mirror neurons play a crucial role in feeding.	☐
Open space in mouth, throat, and nasal areas continues to increase through cranial and jaw growth, as well as the shrinking of the sucking pads between 4 and 6 months.	☐
Baby develops increased lip control and movement between 4 and 6 months.	☐
Baby begins to learn to use jaw, lip, cheek, and tongue muscles independently.	☐
Discriminative mouthing begins: baby explores appropriate toys and fingers throughout his or her mouth between 5 and 9 months.	☐
Teeth begin to come in with increased chewing and biting experiences as well as discriminative mouthing around 6 months.	☐
Appropriate intraoral pressure is maintained through the valving of structures (mouth structures come together and move apart like the closing and opening of a valve).	☐
Baby has easy nose-breathing.	☐
Mouth is closed during sleep and when mouth is inactive (not feeding, mouthing, or making vocal sounds).	☐
Tongue rests in the roof of the mouth to help maintain the broad palate shape (pacifier or bottle nipple cannot do this, but proper breastfeeding can help keep the broad palate shape).	☐
Baby is free of tethered oral tissues, such as tongue tie.	☐
Baby has a good amount of intentional, supervised tummy or belly time as well as other body positions to support postural control needed for rolling, sitting, feeding, vocalization, etc.	☐

3 TO 6 MONTHS continued	CHECK MARK
FEEDING	
BREASTFEEDING AND BOTTLE-FEEDING	
Suck-swallow-breathe coordination improves between 3 and 4 months.	☐
A sequence of 20 or more sucks occurs without a pause (may see a difference between breast-fed and bottle-fed babies).	☐
Coughing or choking occurs only occasionally between 3 and 4 months.	☐
Baby recognizes the bottle when she sees it between 3 and 4 months.	☐
Baby pats bottle or breast with her hand(s) between 3 and 4 months.	☐
Baby can bring an object to her mouth around 4 months.	☐
Baby places his or her hands on the bottle around 4½ months and holds the bottle with his or her hand or hands around 5½ months; baby's body is held/positioned upright at 45+ degree angle to the horizon (not lying down) while bottle-feeding to keep liquid from going into the Eustachian tubes.	☐
OPEN CUP- AND STRAW-DRINKING	
Baby is ready to experiment with drinking from an open cup; cup is held by the parent or care provider (between 4 and 6 months).	☐
May see tongue extrusion reflex (tongue coming out to meet the cup or going under cup) when introducing open cup-drinking—this usually resolves as your baby becomes comfortable closing his or her lips on the cup rim between 4 and 6 months.	☐
Baby takes sips from an open cup held by a parent or care provider around 6 months.	☐

3 TO 6 MONTHS continued	CHECK MARK
Baby can also learn to drink from a squeezable bottle with a straw around 6 months.	☐
SPOON- AND HAND-FEEDING	
Baby's mouth is ready for a soft baby cookie, baby cereal, as well as pureed and well-mashed foods with very small, soft lumps from a spoon around 6 months.	☐
May initially see tongue extrusion reflex (tongue pushing food out), but this resolves as your baby becomes comfortable with closing his or her lips on the spoon (around 6 months).	☐
Baby learns to hold the tongue and jaw still in anticipation of the spoon around 6 months.	☐
Baby bites and chews on soft baby cookies, using rhythmic bite reflex or munching, when cookie is held along with parent or care provider (around 6 months).	☐
Baby may use diagonal rotary chewing pattern if food is placed on the side gum surfaces around 6 months.	☐
Baby sucks to swallow food and liquid around 6 months.	☐

Development (3 to 6 months)

A lot of changes are happening in your baby's structures and feeding abilities between 3 and 6 months of age. You will see his or her tongue extrusion and Babkin reflexes fade at 3 to 4 months of age. You will also see less of his rooting reflex at 3 to 6 months. These reflexes seem to be disappearing, but reflexes do not really disappear. The movement area of your baby's brain is developing and taking control, so the reflex is not needed. Therefore, your baby may locate the breast without rooting. The third lips (the slight gum swelling during feeding that seemed to help with the breast or bottle latch) will also seem to disappear.

Between 4 and 6 months of age, the gag reflex will be stimulated further back on your baby's tongue. New mouthing and feeding experiences allow this to occur. Your baby will mouth and chew on appropriate toys such as Beckman TriChews by ARK Therapeutic, a Baby Grabber by ARK Therapeutic, Chewy Tubes' Baby Mouth Toys, or other appropriate baby mouth toys made from approved materials.

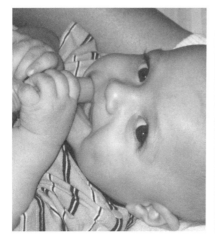

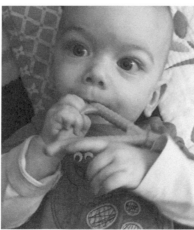

Photo 1.3: *Anthony (4 months) bites on and mouths an Infa-Dent brush during oral massage. Cannon (6.5 months) bites on a Beckman TriChew on his own. Both boys have a nice hand-mouth connection.*

Breastfed babies have a particular advantage when it comes to the integration of the gag reflex. If your baby is breastfeeding properly, the breast is drawn deeply into your baby's mouth, which helps the gag become located further back on the tongue. As your baby gains control over his mouth space and movement, the gag reflex does not need to occur as far forward on the tongue. However, it will still help protect your baby from items too large to swallow. Of course, you will be careful to give your baby appropriately sized mouth toys and foods when you introduce them.

Mirror neurons (where your baby mirrors what you do) play a crucial role in feeding and other activities. Therefore, it's essential to be a good role model for your baby, beginning at birth. This includes the movements you make, what you say, and your social interactions. When you give foods and liquids to your baby (beginning around 6 months), it's very important you eat and drink along with him as much as possible. Your baby understands more than you think, so you will want to be a good role model as you talk and socialize with him. You are helping him set down life-long eating, drinking, and interaction patterns.

Between 5 and 9 months of age, your baby will explore appropriate toys and his own fingers throughout his mouth. He may use his mouth like a *third hand* for this exploration. This leads to good oral discrimination needed for eating, drinking, and ultimately speaking. According to Suzanne Evans Morris and Marsha Dunn Klein, the mouth and hands have the most sensory receptors per square inch in the human body.[32]

Additionally, your baby's phasic bite reflex comes under control with proper biting and chewing experiences between 5 and 9 months. Around 6 months of age, your baby's teeth may begin to come in as he has appropriate biting and chewing experiences. The processes of taking bites and chewing help develop the jaw, lips, cheeks, and tongue muscles, as well as assist in the appearance of teeth. In my experience, babies who don't chew and bite on suitable toys and foods are often late in tooth development and have increased jaw, lip, cheek, and tongue problems.

During the 3- to 6-month period, the space within your baby's mouth, throat, and nasal areas increases. Your baby's palate (mouth roof), nasal, sinus, and throat areas are developing. There is expanding open space in your baby's mouth because his skull and jaw are growing and his sucking pads are getting smaller (between 4 and 6 months). Additionally, your baby will have increasing lip and cheek control and movement. Lips and cheeks work together in feeding and in speech.

Your baby's mouth structures are learning to move independently of one another over time. For example, the tongue, lips, and cheeks begin moving independently of the jaw. Therapists call this *dissociation*. This process allows valving within the mouth where appropriate mouth structures come together and move apart like the closing and opening of a valve.

Through this valving, your baby will learn to control the pressure changes within his mouth. Therapists call this *intraoral pressure*. The mouth, throat, esophagus, voice box, and respiratory system are really systems with valves and pressure changes. You will also see your baby move his mouth just enough for the activity in which he is engaged. Therapists call this *grading* of movement. The processes of dissociation, grading, and valving allow the development of mature eating, drinking, and ultimately speaking skills.

As your baby's mouth, nose, and throat areas continue to grow and change, he should have easy nose-breathing. His mouth should be closed during sleep and when his mouth is inactive or quiet (not feeding, mouthing hands or toys, or making vocal sounds). His tongue should rest in the roof of his mouth to help maintain the broad palate shape. His mouth should be free of tethered oral tissues, such as tongue tie. He also requires a good amount of intentional, supervised tummy or belly time, as well as other body positions to create the foundation for the postural control required for all body movement, including feeding and vocal development.

Photo 1.4: *Mouth, airway, and facial features change significantly in the first 6 months of life due to jaw and other growth. Around 6 months, your child is ready to begin learning culturally appropriate feeding skills.*

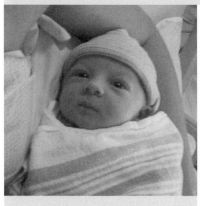

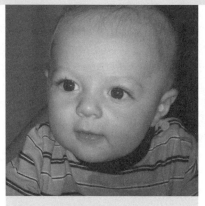

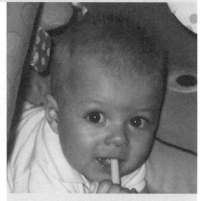

Anthony at birth   *Anthony at 4 months*   *Anthony at 6 months*

Feeding (3 to 6 months)

At 3 to 4 months of age, your baby now recognizes the breast or bottle when he or she sees it. He will pat the bottle or breast with his hand(s). Your baby's suck-swallow-breathe coordination is improving substantially. You will hear only occasional coughing if your baby loses control of this coordination. He will suck 20 or more times without a pause from the breast or bottle. This may be slightly different for breastfed versus bottle-fed babies. See section on breastfeeding and bottle-feeding differences.

Your baby puts his hands on the bottle around 4½ months and holds the bottle around 5½ months of age while being held or positioned upright at an angle of 45+ degrees to the horizon (not lying down). His mouth and digestive system are getting ready for baby cereals, pureed and well-mashed foods, and soft baby cookies by 6 months. Check with your child's pediatrician about when to begin complementary foods with your baby. There are iron-fortified baby cereals if your child's pediatrician says your baby needs extra iron.

The World Health Organization (WHO) recommends exclusive breastfeeding during the first 6 months of life for optimum infant health, growth, and development. Breastfeeding may continue until age 2 or beyond in some cases. Nutritious, appropriate, and complementary foods are introduced around age 6 months.[33][34] These guidelines are similar to recommendations from the American Academy of Pediatrics (AAP). However, at times, pediatricians may recommend feeding complementary foods prior to 6 months for specific children if they are living in developed countries with a safe food supply.

Your baby is ready to experiment with drinking from an open cup (using breast milk or formula) between 4 and 6 months as you hold the cup. You may see the tongue extrusion reflex (tongue coming out to meet the cup or going under the cup) when introducing open cup-drinking, but this resolves as your baby becomes comfortable closing his lips on the cup rim. By 6 months, your baby can take sips from an open cup held by you.

Additionally, your baby is usually sitting up by 6 months. This places him in a good position for eating from a spoon, as well as and drinking from an open cup or flexible squeeze straw bottle. Baby cereals or pureed foods can be given with a spoon or an open cup as your baby is ready to learn these skills. In fact, appropriate pureed foods or baby cereals thinned with water can help you teach open cup- and straw-drinking around 6 months. Straw-drinking is initially taught using a squeezable bottle with a straw. We will discuss spoon-feeding, open cup- and straw-drinking, as well as other feeding processes extensively in Chapter 4.

Your baby's mouth is ready for baby cereal, as well as pureed and well-mashed foods with very small, soft lumps from a spoon around 6 months. You may initially see the tongue extrusion reflex (tongue pushing food out), but this resolves as your baby becomes comfortable with closing his lips on the spoon. He also learns to hold the tongue and jaw still in anticipation of the spoon around 6 months.

At 5 to 6 months of age, your baby will still use the suck to swallow. The mature, adult-like swallowing pattern (where the tongue tip touches the ridge behind the top front teeth to start the swallow) will begin to be seen around 11 to 12 months of age. With an increase in biting and chewing activities on appropriate mouth toys between 3 and 6 months of age, your baby is ready to bite on a soft baby cookie (such as an arrowroot cookie) by 6 months of age. He will use the rhythmic bite reflex or munching pattern to bite on the cookie, held along with a parent or care provider. If a small piece of cookie or soft, small lump of food is placed on your baby's side gums, you may see some diagonal rotary chewing. This means the jaw is moving sideways and diagonally and then back to center to chew the food.

Circular rotary chewing (when the jaw moves in a circle or tear drop shape) is the way we chew our food as adults. Your child will develop this by 2 to 3 years of age. Even though you have just started giving your baby foods around 6 months of age, he or she is quickly ready to begin foods with small, soft lumps, thickened purees and cereals, and soft baby cookies.

Place a check mark next to the characteristics you see in your baby at 6 to 12 months of age.

6 TO 12 MONTHS	CHECK MARK
DEVELOPMENT	
The involuntary suckling reflex seems to be disappearing between 6 and 12 months.	☐
The gag reflex is located on the back ⅓ of the tongue, secondary to feeding and appropriate mouthing experiences between 6 and 9 months.[35]	☐
Control develops over the transverse (side) tongue reflex between 6 and 8 months.	☐
Transverse (side) tongue reflex seems to be disappearing between 9 and 24 months.	☐
Control of the phasic bite reflex develops between 5 and 9 months, with increasing diagonal rotary jaw movement between 6 and 11 months.	☐
The phasic bite reflex seems to disappear between 9 and 12 months.	☐
The grasp reflex seems to disappear around 8 months.	☐

6 TO 12 MONTHS continued	CHECK MARK
Mirror neurons play a crucial role in feeding.	☐
Bottom 2 front teeth (central incisors) come in between 6 and 10 months.	☐
Top 2 front teeth (central incisors) come in and remove food from bottom lip between 8 and 12 months.	☐
Bottom lateral incisors come in between 10 and 16 months.	☐
Top lateral incisors come in between 9 and 13 months.	☐
Nasal breathing is important at all ages.	☐
FEEDING	
Sucks liquid from breast and/or bottle with up-down tongue and jaw movement between 6 and 9 months.	☐
Long suck, swallow, breathe sequences from the breast and/or bottle between 6 and 12 months.	☐
Learns to manage many different food and liquid textures; relies less on breastfeeding and bottle-feeding between 6 and 12 months. See the Food and Liquid Introduction Checklist in next section for details.	☐
OPEN CUP- AND STRAW-DRINKING	
Drinks from an open cup with wide jaw movements at first between 5 and 7 months.	☐
1 to 3 sucks from open cup with improved jaw control between 6 and 8 months.	☐
Up-down tongue movement during open cup-drinking around 8 months.	☐

6 TO 12 MONTHS continued	CHECK MARK
More than 3 consecutive suck-swallows from open cup between 9 and 15 months. Recessed-lid cup (similar to open cup) may be introduced.	☐
Learns to drink from a straw between 6 and 12 months.	☐
Continuous, consecutive sucks (3 or more) during proper straw-drinking between 6 and 12 months.	☐
SPOON-FEEDING	
Baby looks at the spoon and holds mouth still prior taking food from the spoon between 6 and 7 months.	☐
Upper lip moves forward and downward to remove food from the spoon between 6 and 8 months.	☐
Lower lip moves inward after spoon removal between 6 and 12 months.	☐
Lip closure during swallowing begins around 8 months.	☐
Holds/bangs spoon around 9 months; imitates stirring with spoon around 9½ months.	☐
Up-down tongue movement when sucking food from a spoon around 11 months.	☐
FINGER-FEEDING	
Baby can pick up food pieces with a fist and hold a soft baby cookie or cracker to eat it between 6 and 8 months.	☐
Baby can pass a piece of food from one hand to the other between 8 and 9 months.	☐
Begins to pick up small food pieces with thumb and fingers instead of fist between 9 and 12 months.	☐

6 TO 12 MONTHS continued	CHECK MARK
TAKING BITES AND CHEWING	
Jaw movements when taking bites and chewing begin to match the shape and size of the food around 6 months.	☐
Lip and cheek begin to tighten to keep food in place during chewing on side where food is placed around 6 months.	☐
Lips active with chewing between 6 and 9 months.	☐
Lips move inward slightly when food remains on them; lip corner and cheek move inward on the side of chewing between 8 and 11 months.	☐
Upper lip moves forward and downward during chewing between 8 and 12 months.	☐
Cheeks control and move food between 8 and 18 months; lips and cheeks work together.	☐
Lower lip moves inward while food is removed with upper incisors between 9 and 21 months.	☐
Up-down munching on food between 6 and 9 months.	☐
Baby uses up-down biting and chewing/munching on a soft cookie between 6 and 9 months and on a hard cookie between 6 and 19 months.	☐
Diagonal rotary chewing seen on the side where food is placed between 6 and 9 months.	☐
Controls the bite on a soft cookie between 7 and 12 months and on a hard cookie between 11 and 24 months.	☐
The tongue moves up-and-down with the jaw but begins to move toward small pieces of food on the side gums with a rolling or shifting motion between 6 and 9 months.	☐
The tongue begins to move independently from the jaw during sucking between 7 and 11 months and with food transfer from the center of tongue to both sides of the mouth between 7 and 12 months.	☐

Development (6 to 12 months)

Many changes occur in your child's skills during the 6- to 12-month period. The involuntary suckling reflex your baby had at birth seems to disappear between 6 and 12 months. Between 6 and 9 months, your baby's gag reflex matures and is located on the back ⅓ of the tongue. This occurred through breastfeeding; the appropriate mouthing of toys, objects, and fingers; as well as your baby's exposure to many new feeding experiences. Your own gag reflex should be on the back ¼ of your tongue.

Your baby develops control over the transverse (side) tongue reflex between 6 and 8 months, but it may not seem to disappear until 9 to 24 months. Between 5 and 9 months, your baby develops control over her phasic bite reflex as she takes bites of food and increasingly uses diagonal rotary chewing. The phasic bite reflex seems to disappear between 9 and 12 months. You notice most of the mouth reflexes are coming under control and seeming to disappear as your baby is using the mouth intentionally for exploring appropriate objects and toys, eating, drinking, and vocalizing (cooing, babbling). Your baby's grasp reflex also seems to disappear around 8 months.

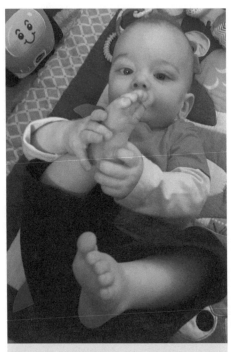

Photo 1.5: *Cannon (6.5 months) thinks toes are good for mouthing too!*

Mirror neurons play a crucial role in feeding and other activities. Therefore, it's essential to be a good role model for your baby beginning at birth. This includes the movements you make as well as your social interactions. When you feed your baby, it's important you have a meal or snack along with her as often as possible. Family meals are vital experiences for you and your baby. Your baby understands more than you think, so you will want to be a good role model as you talk and socialize with her. You are helping her develop life-long interaction, eating, and drinking patterns. I've noticed clinically children often do not want to participate in activities when others are not doing the activities along with them. This seems to begin around 1 year of age.

Teeth come in during this period as your baby is exploring, biting, and chewing on mouth toys, as well as taking bites of and chewing food. Babies need to take bites and chew to get teeth. The bottom 2 front teeth (central incisors) usually emerge between 6 and 10 months. The top 2 front teeth (central incisors) come in and begin to remove food from the bottom lip between 8 and 12 months. The bottom lateral incisors erupt between 10 and 16 months, with the top lateral incisors erupting between 9 and 13 months. Nasal breathing is important at all ages.

Feeding (6 to 12 months)

Your baby will continue to drink liquid from the breast and/or bottle with long periods of coordinated sucking, swallowing, and breathing. Her jaw and tongue should move up-and-down during sucking (not front-back). She will also learn to manage many different food and liquid textures during this time. See the Food and Liquid Introduction Checklist in the next section for details.

You will introduce the open cup to your baby between 5 and 7 months of age by giving her single sips of liquid (beginning with breast milk or formula). Between 6 and 8 months of age, your child can sequence 1 to 3 sucks from an open cup. She has up-down tongue and jaw movement when drinking from an open cup around 8 months. Between 9 and 15 months, she can coordinate 3 or more sucks and swallows from the open cup. During this time a recessed-lid cup (similar to an open cup but with a lid) may be introduced. Between 6 and 12 months, your child can also learn to drink from a straw, beginning with a squeezable bottle containing a straw. Specific information on teaching and learning open cup- and straw-drinking is found in Chapter 4. *Sippy* (or spouted) cups are *not recommended*. Children tend to drink from these in a manner similar to bottle-drinking. The spout holds the tongue tip down in the mouth while a mature swallowing pattern (beginning around 11 months of age) requires the tongue tip to move upward. These types of cups also tend to leave liquid in the mouth which may contribute to tooth decay.[36][37][38][39]

Your baby can also learn spoon-feeding beginning around 6 months of age. She will look at the spoon and make her mouth quiet or still when the spoon approaches her mouth between 6 and 7 months. Between 6 and 8 months of age, your baby's upper lip will move forward and downward to remove food from the spoon. Between 6 and 12 months of age, her lower lip will move inward after the spoon is removed from her mouth. Lip closure for swallowing can begin around 8 months of age. She may hold and bang a spoon around 9 months and imitate stirring around 9½ months. Up-down tongue movement (independent of jaw movement) can be seen around 11 months of age when she sucks food from the spoon. This is the beginning of the mature adult-like swallowing pattern.

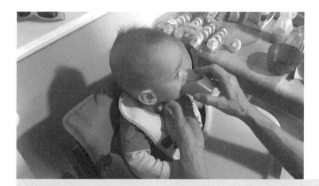 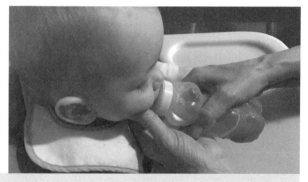

Photo 1.6: *Cannon (6.5 months) learns to drink from a small, pink cut-out cup with a little jaw support and from a Talk-Tools squeezable straw-bottle with gentle cheek support.*

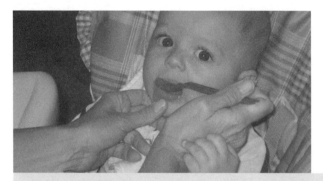 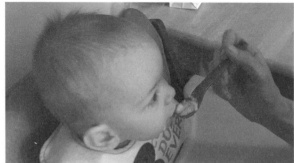

Photo 1.7: *Anthony and Cannon learn to eat from a spoon around 6 months. Anthony receives some jaw support and has a good hand-mouth connection. Cannon makes wonderful eye contact with the feeder. A side spoon-feeding method taught by Sara Rosenfeld-Johnson and Lori Overland is used with both boys.*

Your baby will pick up food pieces in her fist and feed herself a soft baby cookie between 6 and 8 months. By 8 to 9 months, she can pass food from one hand to the other. She can also begin picking up small pieces of food with her thumb and fingers instead of her fist between 9 and 12 months.

Around 6 months, your baby's jaw movements begin to match the shape and size of food pieces when she takes bites and chews them. Her lips and cheeks will also tighten to keep food in place during chewing. Her lips will become active during chewing between 6 and 8 months. Her lips will also move inward when food is left on them. Her lip and cheek corners will move inward on the side she is chewing between 8 and 11 months. Her upper lip will move downward and forward when chewing between 8 and 12 months. Between 8 and 18 months, her cheeks can be seen to control and move food as her lips and cheeks work together. Her lower lip will move inward while food is removed by her upper incisor teeth between 9 and 21 months.

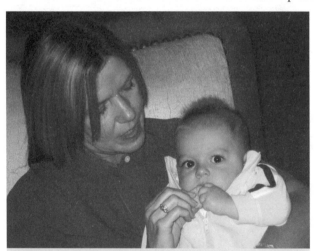

Photo 1.8: *Anthony (6 months) eats a soft arrowroot cookie with a good hand-mouth connection. In many Westernized cultures, feeding at 6 months includes safe hand-held foods, open cup and straw drinking, as well as spoon-feeding. Other cultures may primarily use their hands or other utensils.*

Your baby may use an up-down munching pattern on food between 6 and 9 months. For example, she may munch on a soft cookie between 6 and 9 months and on a hard cookie between 6 and 19 months. She can control her bite on a soft cookie between 7 and 12 months and on a hard cookie between 1 and 24 months. Her tongue initially moves up-and-down with her jaw but begins to move toward small pieces of food placed on the side gums between 6 and

9 months. Her tongue will begin to move independently of her jaw when sucking between 7 and 11 months. This is what therapists call *dissociation*, where one structure moves separately from another. She will also begin to move food from the center of her tongue to each side of her mouth between 7 and 12 months. This is the beginning of what therapists call *tongue lateralization*, a fundamental process for food manipulation and management.

Place a check mark next to the characteristics you see in your child at 12 to 18 months of age.

12 TO 18 MONTHS	CHECK MARK
DEVELOPMENT	
Jaw, lips/cheeks, and tongue continue to learn to move independently of one another.	☐
Different parts of each structure also learn to move separately (as examples, the tip of the tongue begins to move independently of the rest of tongue; each lip corner/cheek contracts independently from rest of lips).	☐
The tongue extrusion (forward) reflex is seen less and less, seems to be disappearing (12 to 18 months); the transverse (side) tongue reflex is seen less and less, seems to be disappearing between 9 and 24 months.	☐
Gains control of swallowing reflex around 18 months.	☐
Mirror neurons play a crucial role in feeding.	☐
Bottom lateral incisors come in between 10 and 16 months.	☐
Top lateral incisors come in between 9 and 13 months.	☐
Bottom first molars come in between 14 and 18 months.	☐
Top first molars come in between 13 and 19 months.	☐
Bottom cuspids/canines come in between 17 and 23 months.	☐

12 TO 18 MONTHS continued	CHECK MARK
Top cuspids/canines come in between 16 and 22 months.	☐
FEEDING	
Tongue moves food from center to side while jaw stays in center between 12 and 36 months.	☐
Beginning around 11 to 12 months, the tip of the tongue intermittently rises to the ridge behind the top front teeth to initiate the swallow (may be seen as early as 7 to 8 months).	☐
Lower lip moves inward and top front teeth remove food from the bottom lip between 9 and 21 months.	☐
Lip corners and cheeks move in to control where food goes in the mouth between 8 and 18 months.	☐
Lips may close during the swallow.	☐
CUP- AND STRAW-DRINKING	
More than 3 continuous, consecutive sucks and swallows when drinking from an open cup, a cup with a recessed lid, or a straw between 9 and 15 months.	☐
If cup has handle(s), baby holds handle(s) when drinking around 12 months.	☐
Holds open cup, and drinks with some spillage around 12 months.	☐
Ready for weaning from bottle between 12 and 15 months; mostly drinks from recessed-lid cup, open cup, or straw cup.	☐
May bite on open cup rim for jaw stability between 11 and 24 months.	☐

12 TO 18 MONTHS continued	CHECK MARK
SPOON-FEEDING	
Begins to feed self with spoon, but may turn it over on the way to the mouth between 12 and 14 months.	☐
Scoops food with spoon, but may spill some when bringing it to the mouth between 15 and 18 months.	☐
FINGER-FEEDING	
Child can finger-feed around 12 months.	☐
Can pick up small food pieces with thumb and index finger between 12 and 15 months.	☐
Puts food pieces into a bowl between 12 and 15 months.	☐
TAKING BITES AND CHEWING	
Can easily bite through a soft cookie with the front teeth; may use munching pattern on hard cookie between 6 and 19 months; controls the bite on a hard cookie between 11 and 24 months.	☐
Eats chopped up table food and very soft meats, such as stewed chicken and ground meat. See Food and Liquid Introduction Checklist in next section for details.	☐
Has coordinated diagonal rotary jaw movement when chewing.	☐
Lips are active during chewing.	☐
Keeps food and saliva in mouth when chewing between 12 and 36 months.	☐

Development (12 to 18 months)

Your child's feeding skills become increasingly refined during the 12- to 18-month period. Her jaw, lips, cheeks, and tongue continue to learn to move independently of one another. Parts of each structure also learn to move separately. As examples, the tongue tip begins to move independently of the rest of the tongue and each lip corner/cheek contracts independently from the rest of the lips. These processes are important for the development of the mature swallowing pattern and effective food manipulation used throughout life.

The tongue extrusion (forward) and the transverse (side) tongue reflexes are seen less. Your child will gain control of her swallowing reflex around 18 months of age. She will also develop a number of teeth during this period. The bottom lateral incisors come in between 10 and 16 months, and the top lateral incisors come in between 9 and 13 months. Her bottom first molars will come in between 14 and 18 months, and her top first molars will come in between 13 and 19 months. Her cuspids (or canines) will come in a bit later, with the bottom cuspids coming in between 17 and 23 months and the top cuspids coming in between 16 and 22 months.

Feeding (12-18 months)

Between 12 and 36 months, your child's tongue will move food from the center of the mouth to the side for chewing while her jaw remains in the center. Beginning around 11 to 12 months, the tip of her tongue rises intermittently to the ridge behind her top front teeth to start her swallow. This is where you begin to see the mature swallow developing.

During the 9- to 21-month period, your child will move the lower lip inward, so the top front teeth can remove food from the lower lip. Your child's lip corners and cheeks move inward to control food placement in the mouth between 8 and 18 months, and her lips may close during the swallow.

Open cup- and straw-drinking continue to develop. Between 9 and 15 months, your child can take more than 3 continuous, consecutive swallows from an open cup, a cup with a recessed lid,

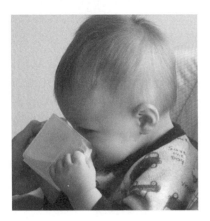 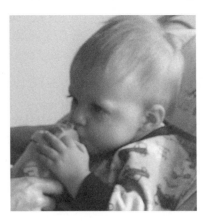

Photo 1.9: *Anthony (12 months) is drinking from a recessed-lid cup with handles (on left) and a regular straw cup (on right). Small regular straw cups are now available, but they are often labeled for older children. A 12-month old can usually drink from a straw cup.*

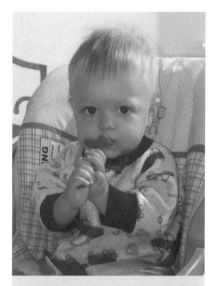

Photo 1.10: *Anthony (12 months) is learning to self-feed with a flat spoon and lip bumper. He continues to have a wonderful hand-mouth connection.*

or a straw. Sippy (spouted) cups are *not recommended.* Children tend to drink from these in a manner similar to bottle drinking. Spouts can also inhibit the development of the mature swallowing pattern, which begins around 11 months of age. These types of cups also tend to leave liquid in the mouth which may contribute to tooth decay. [40][41][42][43]

Around 12 months, your child can hold cup handles when drinking. She can also hold an open cup with some spillage. She is ready to be weaned from the bottle between 12 and 15 months, while breastfeeding may continue. Ask your child's pediatrician to help guide you in the weaning process. Your child will be drinking most of her liquid from a recessed-lid cup, open cup, or straw cup during this progression. When drinking from the open cup, she may bite on the cup rim for jaw stability between 11 and 24 months.

Between 12 and 14 months, your child will begin to feed herself with a spoon. She may turn the spoon over on the way to her mouth. During the 15- to 18-month period, your child will scoop her food with a spoon, although she may still spill some food when bringing it to her mouth.

Children can finger-feed around 12 months. Between 12 and 15 months, your child will pick up small food pieces with her thumb and index finger tips. You will also see her put food pieces into a bowl.

During the 12- to 18-month period, your child will bite through a soft cookie or cracker with ease. Between 6 and 19 months, your child will use an up-down munching pattern on a hard cookie. She learns to control her bite on a hard cookie between 11 and 24 months. Also, during the 12- to 18-month period, your child will eat chopped table food and very soft meats such as stewed chicken or ground meat. She will use a coordinated diagonal rotary chew, and her lips will be active as she chews. Between 12 and 36 months, she will learn to keep food and saliva in her mouth while chewing. See the Food and Liquid Introduction Checklist in the next section for details.

Mirror neurons play a crucial role in feeding and other activities. Therefore, it's essential to be a good role model for your baby beginning at birth. This includes the movements you make as well as your social interactions. When you feed your baby, it's important you eat along with her as much as possible. Additionally, your baby understands more that you think, so you will want to be a good role model as you talk and socialize with her. You are helping her develop life-long eating, drinking, and interaction patterns.

Place a check mark next to the characteristics you see in your child at 18 to 24 months of age.

18 TO 24 MONTHS	CHECK MARK
DEVELOPMENT	
Good control of swallowing by 18 months, but swallowing reflex hopefully continues throughout life; typical swallow continues to mature between 7 and 36 months.	☐
Gag reflex usually remains throughout life on back ¼ of the tongue.	☐
Tongue protrusion (forward) reflex seen less and less, seems to be disappearing between 12 and 18 months; transverse (side) tongue reflex seen less and less, seems to be disappearing between 9 and 24 months.	☐
Palmomental reflex can be seen into adulthood in some individuals.	☐
Mirror neurons play a crucial role in feeding.	☐
Lower canines, or cuspids, come in between 17 and 23 months.	☐
Upper canines, or cuspids, come in between 16 and 22 months.	☐
Lower first molars come in between 14 and 18 months.	☐
Upper first molars come in between 13 and 19 months.	☐
Lower second molars come in between 23 and 31 months.	☐
Upper second molars come in between 25 and 33 months.	☐
Jaw, lips, cheeks, and tongue continue to learn to move independently of one another.	☐

18 TO 24 MONTHS continued	CHECK MARK
Different parts of each structure continue to learn to move independently (tongue tip moving separately from rest of tongue; each lip corner and cheek contracting independently of rest of lips).	☐
FEEDING	
Tries to feed Mom, Dad, or care provider between 18 and 21 months.	☐
Tries to wash and dry hands between 18 and 21 months.	☐
Lower lip moves inward while food is removed with upper incisors between 9 and 21 months.	☐
Lip closure when swallowing solid foods around 18 months, but varies.	☐
Jaw stability increases significantly between 18 and 36 months.	☐
Can easily move tongue to place and collect food for chewing and swallowing.	☐
Mature, adult-like tongue tip elevation to start the swallow, which began around 11 to 12 months, is becoming well established; coughing or choking is seldom seen.	☐
CUP- AND STRAW-DRINKING	
May still bite down on open cup rim to stabilize jaw between 11 and 24 months.	☐
Can drink from an open cup, recessed-lid cup, and straw.	☐
Uses lips actively when drinking from an open cup; can hold an open cup with 1 hand (between 20 to 22 months) without spilling by 24 months.	☐

18 TO 24 MONTHS continued	CHECK MARK
SPOON- OR FORK-FEEDING	
By 24 months, has palm up when bringing spoon or fork to mouth (parent continues to stab food for child with the fork).	☐
TAKING BITES AND CHEWING	
May use up-down munching pattern on a hard cookie between 6 and 19 months; controls bite on a hard cookie between 11 and 24 months.	☐
Eats chopped foods including many meats and raw vegetables between 18 and 21 months.	☐
By 24 months, can manage most foods in bite-sized pieces cut by parent or created by taking bites.	☐
Keeps food and saliva in mouth when chewing between 12 and 36 months.	☐
Tongue moves food from center to side while jaw stays in the center between 12 and 36 months.	☐
Tongue tip moves independently of the jaw to clear lips or inner cheek areas between 18 and 36 months.	☐
Tongue moves food from one side of the mouth to the other between 21 and 36 months.	☐
Circular or tear-drop shaped chewing (between 24 and 36 months).	☐
Can chew with closed lips.	☐

Development (18 to 24 months)

Your child will have good control of swallowing by 18 months. Swallowing typically matures between 7 and 36 months. Both the swallowing and gag reflexes hopefully remain throughout life. The gag reflex is usually on the back ¼ of the tongue. By 18 months, the tongue protrusion (forward) reflex is usually not seen, and the transverse (side) tongue reflex is seen less and less. The palmomental reflex can be seen into adulthood in some individuals.

Most of your child's primary teeth will come in by 33 months. The lower canines, or cuspids, come in between 17 and 23 months, while the upper canines, or cuspids, come in between 16 and 22 months. The lower first molars come in between 14 and 18 months, while the upper first molars come in between 13 and 19 months. The lower second molars come in between 23 and 31 months, while the upper second molars come in between 25 and 33 months.

Feeding (18 to 24 months)

By 24 months of age, your child's jaw, lips, cheeks, and tongue are working independently of one another. This allows your child to eat and drink like you and me. Between 18 and 21 months, your child may try to feed you. She may also try to wash and dry her hands. In my experience, I've seen this begin as early as 1 year of age. Children like to do what they see others doing.

As you know, mirror neurons play a crucial role in feeding and other activities. Therefore, it's essential to be a good role model for your baby beginning at birth. This includes the movements you make as well as your social interactions. When you feed your child, it's important you eat along with him or her as much as possible. Family meals are crucial for good feeding development. Additionally, your child understands more than you think, so you will want to be a good role model as you talk and socialize with him. You are helping him develop life-long eating, drinking, and interaction patterns.

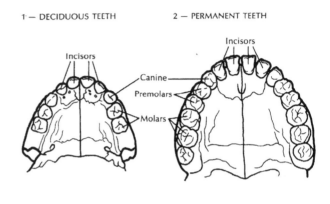

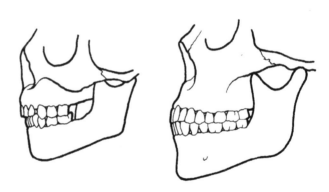

Illustration 3-27
Distribution of Deciduous and Permanent Teeth

Figure 1.2: *Jaw, tooth, and palate development go together. The roof of the mouth should maintain a broad "U" shape throughout life. The deciduous (primary) teeth come in between 6 and 33 months. Chewing from an early age is vital for tooth and jaw development. It is also crucial that the tooth buds for all permanent teeth be present in the gums. Reprinted from* Craniosacral Therapy II: Beyond the Dura *by John E. Upledger, p. 192, with permission of Eastland Press.*

In feeding, your child's lower lip moves inward while food is removed with his upper incisor teeth between 9 and 21 months. He may close his lips when swallowing solid foods around 18 months of age, but this varies. His jaw stability

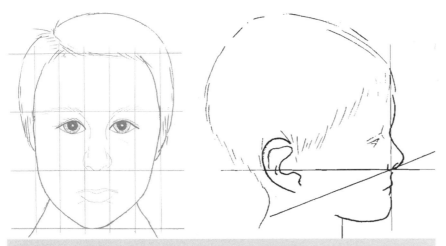

Figure 1.3: *Significant head, jaw, and airway growth occur in the first 2 years of life. This results in balanced facial features. This growth, along with good overall body development, leads to adult-like eating, drinking, swallowing, and speaking. Drawings developed by Artist Anthony Fotia, Sr for Diane Bahr who granted permission for their use. Dimensions suggested by Char Boshart in her book* Oral-Facial Illustrations and Reference Guide *(2013).*

increases significantly between 18 and 36 months. Jaw stability is crucial for eating, drinking, and speaking because the lip, cheek, and tongue muscles are attached to the jaw. So, if the jaw isn't working well, then it's difficult for the lips, cheeks, and tongue to work well. It's also true that if the tongue is tied, it's difficult for the jaw and tongue to grow and work properly.

During the 18- to 24-month period, your child can easily move his tongue to place and collect food for chewing and swallowing. The mature, adult-like tongue tip elevation to start the swallow, which began around 11 to 12 months, is becoming well established, so coughing or choking are seldom seen. When open cup-drinking, your child may still bite down on the cup rim to stabilize the jaw between 11 and 24 months. He will use his lips actively when drinking from an open cup. He can hold an open cup with 1 hand around 20 to 22 months and without spilling by 24 months. He can drink from an open cup, recessed-lid cup, and straw. By 24 months, your child will have his palm up when bringing the spoon or fork to his mouth. However, you will still stab food for him with the fork.

Between 6 and 19 months, your child may use an up-down munching pattern on a hard cookie, but he will learn to control his bite on a hard cookie between 11 and 24 months. He will eat chopped foods, including many meats and raw vegetables between 18 and 21 months. By 24 months, he can manage most foods in bite-sized pieces cut by you or created as he takes appropriately sized bites of food. See the Food and Liquid Introduction Checklist in the next section for details.

Between 12 and 36 months, he will learn to keep food and saliva in his mouth when chewing, and his tongue will move food from center to side while his jaw stays in the center of his mouth. Therapists call this *tongue and jaw dissociation* and *tongue lateralization*. His tongue tip will move independently of his jaw to clear his lips or inner cheek areas of food between 18 and 36 months. His tongue will also move food from one side of his mouth to the other between 21 and 36 months. By 24 to 36 months of age, he will have circular or tear-drop shaped chewing like you and me. Additionally, he can chew with closed lips.

Food and Liquid Introduction Checklist: Birth to 24 Months

Now you know the mechanics of feeding. Here are some literature-based guidelines for introducing foods and liquids. [44] [45] [46] [47] Discuss this process with your child's pediatrician.

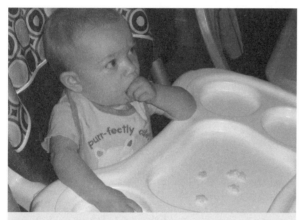

Photo 1.11a: *Rylee is finger feeding baby crackers at 7.5 months.*

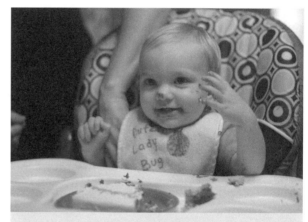

Photo 1.11b: *For her first birthday Rylee says, "Let me get my hands into that delicious cake!"*

Place a check mark next to the foods and liquids your child is eating and drinking.

BIRTH TO 24 MONTHS	CHECK MARK
BIRTH TO 6 MONTHS: BREAST MILK OR INFANT FORMULA	
No extra water normally needed as breast milk and formula usually have plenty of water. A pediatrician may recommend extra water for babies living in hot, dry climates. Boil water for 3 minutes and cool for children under 6 months. Consult your child's pediatrician as *too much water can harm small babies.*[48]	☐
6 MONTHS (UNLESS ADVISED OTHERWISE BY YOUR CHILD'S PEDIATRICIAN)	
Fortified baby cereal mixed with breast milk or formula to start.	☐
Non-wheat cereals, such as oat.	☐

BIRTH TO 24 MONTHS continued	CHECK MARK
Pureed fruits and vegetables.	☐
Sips of water (boiled for 3 minutes and cooled), formula or breast milk from an open cup held by you.	☐
Soft baby cookie held by you and baby, such as *non-wheat* arrowroot or rice.	☐
Breast milk or formula from the breast or bottle, allowing baby to self-limit.	☐
6 TO 8 MONTHS	
Milled, blended, or well-mashed vegetables and fruits (well-cooked with small, soft lumps).	☐
Wheat-free soft cookies, biscuits, and crackers; teething biscuits.	☐
Cooked rice (sticky).	☐
Sips of water, formula, or breast milk from an open- or straw-cup.	☐
Breast milk or formula from breast or bottle, allowing baby to self-limit.	☐
7 TO 10 MONTHS	
Chopped, cooked fruits and vegetable (includes canned fruits but no citrus).	☐
Soft cheese.	☐
Mashed, cooked beans or tofu.	☐

BIRTH TO 24 MONTHS continued	CHECK MARK
Wheat and corn products (such as bread, toast, soft tortilla strips, crackers, dry cereals without sugar, or well-cooked pasta).	☐
Sips of water, formula, or breast milk from an open- or straw-cup.	☐
Breast milk or formula from breast or bottle, allowing baby to self-limit.	☐
9 TO 12 MONTHS	
Soft, cut-up cooked foods and safe, soft, cut-up uncooked foods (such as bananas, skinned peaches, peeled avocado, etc.); introduce citrus slowly.	☐
Cooked fruit or vegetable strips.	☐
Soft, chopped meats (such as stewed chicken, no bone; ground meat; no fish).	☐
Casseroles with noodles, pasta, or rice.	☐
Bread, toast, crackers, dry cereal without sugar (no chocolate).	☐
Eggs (yolks at 9 months, whites at 12 months) and cheese (soft cheese strips, cottage cheese, yogurt formulated for babies).	☐
Sips of water, formula, or breast milk from an open, recessed-lid, or straw cup.	☐
Breast milk or formula from breast or bottle, allowing baby to self-limit.	☐
12 TO 18 MONTHS	
Chopped table food (avoid round foods such as whole grapes and hotdog pieces).	☐

BIRTH TO 24 MONTHS continued	CHECK MARK
Soft meats, including fish (no bones).	☐
Cookies and crackers (can bite through).	☐
Drinks of milk, water, very diluted fruit or vegetable juices (if given) from an open, recessed-lid, or straw cup.	☐
Weaning from the bottle; breastfeeding may continue.	☐
18 TO 21 MONTHS	
Chopped table food, including many meats and raw vegetables.	☐
Can bite through a hard cookie or cracker but may struggle a little.	☐
Drinks of milk, water, very diluted fruit or vegetable juices (if given) from an open, recessed-lid, or straw cup.	☐
Weaned from the bottle; breastfeeding may continue.	☐
BY 24 MONTHS	
Can bite through hard cookie with ease.	☐
Can chew with closed lips and uses mature chewing patterns; can manage most foods in bite-sized pieces cut by parent or created by taking bites.	☐
Uses lips when drinking from an open cup (tongue not in or under cup), can hold an open cup with one hand, and does not spill liquid from an open cup.	☐

As you introduce foods to your baby, introduce 1 food at a time. Wait 3 to 4 days before introducing another food. Look for any sensitivity to the food such as wheezing and/or dry cough, apparent stomach pain, excessive burping and/or reflux, diarrhea, or any type of rash. The first time many parents and pediatricians see food sensitivities in some babies is right after birth. The sensitivity is often indicated by excessive spit up and apparent gastrointestinal discomfort. This is one reason pediatricians may have parents try different formulas.

Breastfed babies tend to have fewer food allergies and sensitivities. However, some breastfed babies are sensitive to certain foods or liquids Mom eats or drinks. Pediatricians and lactation consultants (preferably an IBCLC) will often recommend Mom eliminate certain foods from her diet to see if the baby improves. More information on this topic is found in the book *Nobody Ever Told Me (or my Mother) That! Everything from Bottles and Breathing to Healthy Speech Development* by Diane Bahr.

When introducing a new food or liquid, do not expect your child to like the smell, taste, and texture immediately. Think of when you first try a food or liquid, particularly one from another culture. Do you always like foods or liquids when you first taste them? Your baby's food culture has been different than yours from birth, particularly if you are giving him formula. He has been eating basically the same thing every day if he is drinking formula. However, if you are breastfeeding, your baby is getting some different tastes based on what Mom is eating and drinking.

It may take 10 to 15 opportunities or exposures to a new food or liquid for your child to begin to enjoy it. This is an important idea for you to understand because this is where many of our picky or selective eaters seem to start. If you see your baby make a face or spit food (or liquid) out when he first tastes it, this may just mean he is not accustomed to the smell, taste, or texture. Your baby may actually like the food or liquid when given additional opportunities to experience it.

I mentioned smell a couple of times. Smell is an important food and liquid quality. It can tell us if food or liquid is spoiled. Additionally, most people don't want to taste something when they don't like the smell of it. So, let your baby smell foods and liquids as you introduce them, and talk about the wonderful smells of food or liquid. Also, be careful with what you say about food and liquid. Babies understand more language than many people think. They also understand body language and tone of voice. If you don't like a food or liquid, or you comment about your baby disliking a food or liquid, this can become a self-fulfilling prophecy (your baby may not like the food because of messages he is receiving from you or others feeding him). You can be a good role model by eating, drinking, and talking about different foods or liquids with your child. Meals are social experiences.

Once your baby begins eating modified solid food, around 6 months of age, all of his nutritional requirements change. First, you must remember your child's stomach is about as big as his fist. Therefore, your child's portion sizes will be nowhere near your portion sizes. There are many good resources on nutrition. This book is not meant to replace them. Here are some resources on nutrition in addition to the information your child's pediatrician and pediatric registered dietician or nutritionist may provide:

RESOURCES	WEBSITES
Academy of Nutrition and Dietetics	www.eatright.org
American Academy of Pediatrics	www.aap.org and www.healthychildren.org
Ellyn Satter Institute	www.ellynsatterinstitute.org
Nutrition.gov	www.nutrition.gov

Additionally, baby-led weaning has become a popular way to introduce foods to babies. There are now a number of resources discussing the appropriate use of this technique. In my opinion, baby-led weaning, if done properly, can be an important part of the feeding process. However, I don't feel it should be done to the exclusion of other culturally-appropriate feeding techniques and skill development progressions.

For example, both spoon-feeding (if part of a culture) and experiences with a variety of food textures (such a pureed, mashed, and mixed-texture foods) teach important mouth-development skills as you saw in our first two checklists, Feeding and Related Development Checklist: Birth to 24 Months and Food and Liquid Introduction Checklist: Birth to 24 Months. When using baby-led weaning, a number of articles now suggest a modified version to minimize iron deficiency, growth concerns, choking risks, and difficulties with readiness for certain foods.[49] [50] [51] [52]

There are a number of other books on feeding. Here are a few:

- *Adventures in Veggieland: Help Your Kids Learn to Love Vegetables with 100 Easy Activities and Recipes* by Melanie Potock [53]

- *A Sensory Motor Approach to Feeding* by Lori L. Overland and Robyn Merkel-Walsh [54]

- *Baby Self-Feeding: Solid Food Solutions to Create Lifelong, Healthy Eating Habits* by Nancy Ripton and Melanie Potock [55]

- *Baby-led Weaning: The Essential Guide to Introducing Solid Foods and Helping Your Baby Grow Up a Happy and Confident Eater* by Gill Rapley and Tracey Murkett [56]

- *Child of Mine: Feeding with Love and Good Sense* by Ellyn Satter [57]

- *Happy Mealtimes with Happy Kids: How to Teach Your Child about the Joy of Food* by Melanie Potock [58]

- *Helping Your Child with Extreme Picky Eating: A Step-by-Step Guide for Overcoming Selective Eating, Food Aversion, and Feeding Disorders* by Katja Rowell and Jenny McGlothlin [59]

- *How to Get Your Kid to Eat ... But Not Too Much* by Ellen Satter [60]

- *Just Take a Bite: Easy, Effective, Answers to Food Aversion and Eating Challenges* by Lori Ernsperger and Tania Stegen-Hanson [61]

- *Nobody Ever Told Me (or My Mother) That! Everything from Bottles and Breathing to Healthy Speech Development* by Diane Bahr [62]

- *Pre-Feeding Skills: A Comprehensive Resource for Mealtime Development (2nd ed.)* by Suzanne Evans Morris and Marsha Dunn Klein [63]

Intentional, Supervised Tummy/Belly Time to Creeping/Crawling Checklist: A Likely Fundamental Missing Developmental Link (Birth to 7 Months) [64 65 66 67]

Whereas *back-to-sleep* continues to be the *recommend sleeping position* for babies to avoid Sudden Infant Death Syndrome (SIDS), a baby needs to experience *many different body positions* to develop adequate postural control. Good body (or core) development provides the foundation for both large and small body movements (called gross and fine motor skills).

In this section, we explore what may be a missing developmental link in our current child-rearing methods. With the recommendation for back-to-sleep (*which we must follow*), many babies are spending an inordinate amount of time on their backs. With our on-the-go population, babies are also spending a significant amount of time in car seats, infant seats, swings, and other containers. Therefore, many babies are not developing satisfactory postural control needed for both gross and fine motor skill advancement. This may be the reason we are seeing so many motor delays in children who may otherwise be typical. The motor delays include late rolling, sitting, crawling, walking, feeding, speaking, vision use, reading, and writing. These children are filling therapist's caseloads.

Most mammals are vulnerable on their backs, as vital organs are located on the front of the body. However, due to SIDS research, the current recommendation is to have *babies sleep on their backs.*[68 69 70 71] Therefore, parents and care-providers need to make an extra effort to provide supervised, intentional tummy or belly time as well as other appropriate body positions beginning at birth. The period of intentional or supervised tummy or belly time to creeping (belly on floor) and crawling (belly off of floor) is found in the next checklist. In addition to supervised belly or tummy time and other body positions, babies need to spend a good period of time creeping and crawling. These positions and movements seem to support forward jaw growth with the help of gravity, which is essential for mouth and airway development.

Your baby will not be swaddled during supervised, intentional tummy or belly time. Swaddling may calm a very young baby while sleeping on her back. However, it does not allow the movement development which occurs during supervised, intentional belly time and other body positions. Swaddling likely inhibits the startle or Moro reflex, which wakes babies while sleeping on their backs. This may allow them to recover from events such as gastroesophageal reflux or airway problems. Stress hormones may be released along with the startle and may ultimately be related to apparent increases in sleep and attention problems in children.[72][73][74] This may be one reason pacifiers, which tend to calm babies, have been used to reduce reflux and SIDS. Clearly, much more research is needed in this area regarding infants. However, there is increasing research on airway problems and sleep disorders in children.[75][76][77][78][79]

Michelle Emanuel coined the term *intentional tummy time*. She teaches the Tummy Time Method for parents and professionals. Michelle's method helps regulate the nervous system through play and interaction with a baby.

While a number of resources were used for this checklist, a special thank-you goes to Lois Bly, author of *Motor Skills Acquisition in the First Year: An illustrated Guide to Normal Development*[80] and Shirley German Vulpé, author of the *Vulpe Assessment Battery: Developmental Assessment - Revised, Performance Analysis, Individualized Programming for the Atypical Child*.[81] These books are crucial resources for therapists and other professionals. Both authors discuss the importance of the many body positions needed for the development of movement (back time, belly time, side-lying, weight bearing and shifting, which lead to rolling, sitting, creeping, crawling, kneeling, standing, walking, etc.) This, again, is information often unavailable to parents or pediatricians with the level of detail found here.

Place a check mark next the characteristics you see during your child's intentional, supervised tummy or belly time as well as later creeping and crawling. Look at your child's age if full or close to term. Look at his or her adjusted age if born prematurely.

INTENTIONAL, SUPERVISED TUMMY/BELLY TIME	CHECK MARK
DURING INTENTIONAL BELLY TIME AT BIRTH TO 1 MONTH	
Rests head on one side or the other, but can lift and turn head from side-to-side.	☐
Lifts head and chin for a few moments, freeing nose (arms and legs are gathered in or flexed).	☐
Arms are next to the body, elbows are bent at elbow joints, and hands rest by shoulders.	☐
Hips, knees, and ankles are bent with baby's hips up.	☐

INTENTIONAL, SUPERVISED TUMMY/BELLY TIME continued	CHECK MARK
Arms and legs may move in a crawling motion.	☐
May bend and straighten legs with a thrusting motion.	☐
DURING SUPERVISED TUMMY TIME AT 2 TO 3 MONTHS	
Begins to lift head for 5 to 10 seconds in middle or midline around 2 months, and learns to keep head up without bobbing around 3 months.	☐
Begins to push up with arms and lift chest for 1 to 5 seconds around 2 months.	☐
Begins bearing weight on lower arms (forearms) while elbows line up symmetrically with, or are in front of, the shoulders around 3 to 4 months.	☐
May alternate legs when kicking around 2 months.	☐
Legs can be under hips or stretched out around 3 months.	☐
Begins to look up and follow object or person while on belly around 3 months.	☐
DURING INTENTIONAL BELLY TIME AT 4 TO 5 MONTHS	
Lifts and turns head with good control around 3 to 4 months.	☐
Raises head and chest while resting on lower arms (forearms) for several minutes around 4 to 5 months.	☐
Reaches for objects while holding body up with one arm and can bring object to mouth with other hand around 4 months.	☐
Begins to straighten arms and bear weight in shoulders with help from the upper body around 4 months.	☐

INTENTIONAL, SUPERVISED TUMMY/BELLY TIME continued	CHECK MARK
Begins to reach forward with straightened arms and open hands, bearing weight in hands and shoulders with help from the body's core around 5 months.	☐
Brings arms forward to hold and play with object using both hands around 5 months.	☐
Trunk and legs may move in a swimming motion around 3 to 4 months.	☐
Legs may be stretched out or under hips around 4 months, and legs assist with changes in weight bearing around 5 months.	☐
Tries to move objects by kicking them.	☐
Rolls from belly to side and returns to side around 3 to 4 months, and rolls from back to side around 5 months.	☐
DURING SUPERVISED BELLY TIME TO CREEPING/CRAWLING AT 6 TO 7 MONTHS	
Bears weight on lower arms (forearms) around 6 months.	☐
Can support body weight and push body back with arms and hands around 5 to 6 months.	☐
Pushes body up with stretched out arms, bearing weight on heels of hands around 6 months.	☐
Can pivot body using arms, shoulders, and body's core to shift body weight and reach for objects with head and legs lifted around 5 to 6 months.	☐
Can pivot body in a circle using arms, shoulders, core, and legs around 7 months.	☐
Uses arm or leg to reach for object around 5 to 6 months.	☐
Can support body with one lower arm (forearm) and reach for object with other hand around 5 to 6 months.	☐

INTENTIONAL, SUPERVISED TUMMY/BELLY TIME continued	CHECK MARK
Can reach for, grasp, and bring object to mouth while on belly or side around 5 to 6 months.	☐
Has good shoulder and body control for reaching and grasping around 7 months.	☐
Can push up on hands and knees around 6 months.	☐
Can easily move to hands and knees, push up to hands and feet to stand like a bear, creep, and crawl around 7 months.	☐
Can roll from back or side to belly around 5 to 6 months.	☐
Can roll completely from stomach, to back, to stomach around 6 to 7 months.	☐
Can move via pivoting, creeping, or rolling around 6 to 7 months.	☐
Can sit on own with legs in a circle around 6 months, and can move between sitting and creeping or crawling and alternating arms and legs between 7 and 12 months.	☐
Crawling progresses from front-back body movement, to side-to-side weight shift in the body, to diagonal and rotary movement in the body, which then allows for alternating arm and leg movements when crawling.	☐

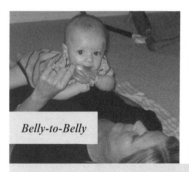

Belly-to-Belly

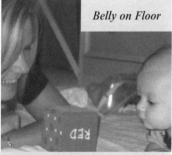

Belly on Floor

Photo 1.12: *Anthony (4 months) is playing in belly time with Diane. The belly-to-belly position is a good way to begin if a child is not accustomed to supervised or intentional belly time.*

During the birth to 1-month period, typically developing, full-term babies of 40 weeks gestation (and most close-to-term babies of 37 to 39 weeks gestation) can rest their heads on one side or the other while supervised on their bellies. They can also lift and turn their heads from side-to-side as long as no extra covers, stuffed animals, etc. are in the way. During supervised, intentional tummy time your baby's arms are next to her body, her elbows

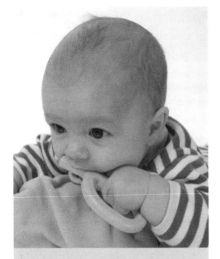

Photo 1.13: *ARK Therapeutic provides (with permission) the photo of a baby in supervised belly time on a slight wedge as he holds and mouths an ARK Baby Grabber (www.ARKTherapeutic.com).*

are bent at the elbow joints, and her hands rest by her shoulders. Her hips, knees, and ankles are bent, and her hips are up. Her arms and legs may move in a crawling motion, or she may bend and straighten her legs with a thrusting motion.

In supervised, intentional tummy time, your baby begins to lift her head for 5 to 10 seconds in midline (middle) around 2 months and learns to keep her head up without bobbing around 3 months. She begins to push up with her arms and raise her chest for 1 to 5 seconds around 2 months of age. She also begins bearing weight on her lower arms (forearms) while her elbows line up with or are in front of her shoulders around 3 to 4 months. She may alternate her legs when kicking around 2 months. Her legs may be under her hips or stretched out around 3 months. Your baby begins to look up and follow objects or people while on her belly around 3 months.

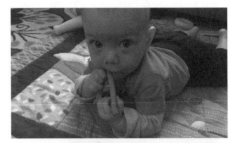

During intentional belly time, your baby will lift and turn her head with good control around 3 to 4 months. She can raise her head and chest for several minutes while resting on her lower arms (forearms) around 4 to 5 months. Your baby will reach for objects while holding her body up with one arm and can bring objects to her mouth with the other around 4 months. She will also shift weight from one arm and shoulder to the other with help from her upper body at this time.

Your baby begins to straighten her arms and bear weight in her shoulders with help from her upper body around 4 months. She also begins to reach forward with straightened arms and open hands while bearing weight in her hands and shoulders with help from her body's core around 5 months. She will bring her arms forward to hold and play with an object using both hands around 5 months.

Around 3 to 4 months, your baby's body and legs may move in a swimming motion. Her legs may be stretched out or under her hips during supervised tummy time around 4 months,

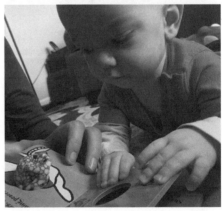

Photo 1.14: *Cannon (6.5 months) chews on a Beckman Tri-Chew and looks at a book in belly time. Supervised, intentional tummy and belly time is vital for overall body, gross motor, and fine motor development. Eating, drinking, speaking, hand-use, and vision-use are fine motor skills used throughout life.*

and her legs will assist with changes in weight bearing throughout her body around 5 months. She may try to move objects by kicking them between 4 to 5 months of age. She will roll from her belly to her side around 3 to 4 months and will roll from her back to her side around 5 months.

As your baby continues supervised, intentional tummy or belly time, she will bear weight on her lower arms (forearms) around 6 months. She can support her body weight and push her body back with her arms and hands around 5 to 6 months. She will also push her body up with stretched-out arms while bearing weight on the heels of her hands around 6 months. Your baby can pivot her body using her arms, shoulders, and core to shift body weight and reach for objects with her head and legs elevated around 5 to 6 months. She can pivot her body in a circle using her arms, shoulders, core, and legs around 7 months. She can use her arms and legs to reach toward objects at 5 to 6 months of age.

Your baby will support her body with one lower arm (forearm) and reach for an object with the other hand around 5 to 6 months of age. She can also reach for, grasp, and bring an object to her mouth while on her belly or side around 5 to 6 months. She has good shoulder and body control for reaching and grasping by 7 months. She can push up on her hands and knees around 6 months. She can easily move up to her hands and knees, push up to hands and feet (bear stand), creep, and crawl around 7 months. Your baby can roll from back or side to belly around 6 months. She can roll completely from her stomach, to her back, to her stomach and can move via pivoting, creeping, and rolling around 6 to 7 months.

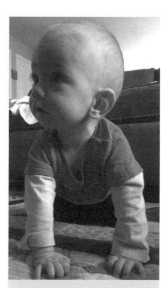

Around 6 months, your baby can sit on her own with her legs in a circle. She can move between sitting and creeping or crawling around 7 months. She will crawl with her belly off of the floor, alternating arm and leg movements between 7 and 12 months. Crawling progresses from front-back body movement on hands and knees to side-to-side weight shifting in the shoulders and hips, to diagonal and rotary movements in the body. This progression allows for alternating arm and leg movements during crawling. If these types of movements do not develop in the body, they are unlikely to develop in the mouth for feeding, which also involves front-back, side-to-side, diagonal, and rotary movements.

Photo 1.15: *Cannon (6.5 months) says, "Look at me Mom! I'm crawling!"*

Mouth and Hand-Mouth Reflex/Response Checklists (Full-Term Baby, 40 Weeks Gestation)

Mouth and hand-mouth reflexes play an important role in feeding development, as seen in the previous Feeding and Related Development Checklist. The following checklists provide you with details regarding these reflexes. Again, parents and care-providers frequently do not have access to this level of detail.

Place a check mark next to the mouth reflexes or responses you see in your child.

MOUTH REFLEXES/RESPONSES PRESENT AT BIRTH 82 83 84 85 86 87 88 89 90 91 92	CHECK MARK
ROOTING REFLEX OR RESPONSE	
Stimulated by touch to the baby's lips or cheeks; her mouth searches for the touch.	☐
Helps the baby find the breast, bottle (if paced, baby-led, bottle-feeding is used), finger, or hand.	☐
Rooting leads to sucking.	☐
Baby begins to gain control over this reflex around 1 month.	☐
It seems to disappear (become integrated by the brain) between 3 and 6 months.	☐
SUCKLING REFLEX OR RESPONSE	
Stimulated when fingers placed into baby's mouth; may also occur with bottle or breast nipple.	☐
Non-nutritive (approximately 2 per second).	☐
Precursor to the nutritive suck established in utero (approximately 1 per second).	☐
Baby begins to gain control over this reflex around 2 to 3 months of age.	☐
It seems to disappear (become integrated by the brain) between 6 and 12 months.	☐
TONGUE EXTRUSION REFLEX OR RESPONSE	

MOUTH REFLEXES/RESPONSES PRESENT AT BIRTH [82 83 84 85 86 87 88 89 90 91 92] continued	CHECK MARK
Touch to baby's tongue or lips stimulates forward tongue motion.	☐
Likely part of the suckling reflex or response.	☐
May protect the baby from ingesting items for which the baby is not ready or are too large.	☐
Baby begins to gain control over this reflex around 3 to 4 months.	☐
It seems to disappear (become integrated by the brain) between 12 and 18 months.	☐
SWALLOWING REFLEX OR RESPONSE	
Triggered as saliva, liquid, and/or food move toward the baby's throat.	☐
Nutritive suck and swallow is approximately 1 per second with good suck-swallow-breathe synchrony (or rhythm).	☐
Baby seems to gain control over the swallow around 18 months.	☐
Important reflex to retain throughout life.	☐
PHASIC BITE REFLEX OR RESPONSE	
Stimulated when firm but gentle pressure is applied to the baby's gums.	☐
The baby opens and closes the jaw in a rhythmic biting pattern (approximately 1 per second).	☐
This reflex works the muscles which raise and lower the jaw; these muscles are used in feeding and babbling.	☐

MOUTH REFLEXES/RESPONSES PRESENT AT BIRTH [82 83 84 85 86 87 88 89 90 91 92] continued	CHECK MARK
Baby begins to gain control of this reflex between 5 and 9 months.	☐
It seems to disappear (become integrated by the brain) between 9 and 12 months.	☐
TRANSVERSE TONGUE REFLEX OR RESPONSE	
Stimulated by touch to either side of the baby's tongue, and the baby's tongue moves toward the touch.	☐
Lateral or sideward tongue movement is ultimately used to place food for chewing and collect food for swallowing.	☐
Baby begins to gain control of this reflex between 6 and 8 months.	☐
It seems to disappear (become integrated by the brain) between 9 and 24 months.	☐
GAG REFLEX OR RESPONSE	
Stimulated by touch to the back ¾ of the baby's tongue at birth.	☐
When stimulated, the baby's mouth opens wide, head may go back, soft palate rises rapidly, and voice box and diaphragm may rise.	☐
It protects the baby from swallowing items that are too large.	☐
Baby begins to gain control of this reflex between 4 and 6 months.	☐
By 6 to 9 months, the gag response is found on back ⅓ of the baby's tongue.	☐
It continues throughout life on the back ¼ of the tongue in most people.	☐

Place a check mark next to the hand-mouth reflexes or responses you see in your child.

HAND-MOUTH REFLEXES AND RESPONSES PRESENT AT BIRTH 93 94 95 96 97	CHECK MARK
PALMOMENTAL REFLEX OR RESPONSE	
Touch to the baby's palms results in wrinkling of the mentalis muscles under the lower lip.	☐
The mentalis muscles evert (turn out) the lower lip for latching.	☐
May be seen into adulthood in some people.	☐
BABKIN REFLEX OR RESPONSE	
Gentle pressure into the base of the baby's palm results in the baby's mouth opening, eyes closing, and head moving forward.	☐
This helps the baby prepare to breastfeed but may also be used in paced (baby-led) bottle-feeding.	☐
This reflex seems to disappear (become integrated by the brain) around 3 to 4 months.	☐
GRASP REFLEX OR RESPONSE	
Stimulated by gently pressing the baby's palm resulting in the baby grasping your finger.	☐
The baby's grasp tightens as she sucks; the baby may also hold on to the feeder's clothing.	☐
This reflex seems to disappear (become integrated by the brain) around 8 months.	☐

Full-term (and close-to-term, 37-39 weeks) babies are born with full-body, mouth, and hand-mouth reflexes. We mentioned the Moro response (a full-body response) in the previous section. However, we are going to discuss reflexes related to feeding in this section. Your child's pediatrician can assess your baby's reflexes.

The rooting reflex or response is stimulated by touching your baby's lips or cheeks. This results in her mouth searching for the touch. The rooting reflex helps your baby find the breast, bottle (if paced, baby-led, bottle-feeding is used), finger, or hand on which to suck. When you watch your baby root, you will see how rooting leads directly to sucking. Your baby will begin to gain control over the rooting reflex around 1 month, and it seems to disappear (or become integrated) between 3 and 6 months. As you know, reflexes are integrated by the brain as the movement area of your baby's brain takes control of movements and a reflex is no longer needed.

Your baby's suckling reflex or response is stimulated when fingers are placed into your baby's mouth. You may also see this with the breast or bottle. It is usually non-nutritive (occurring approximately 2 per second) and used for calming. The suckling response is the precursor to the nutritive suck established in utero (occurring approximately 1 per second). Your baby begins to gain control over this reflex around 2 to 3 months of age. It seems to disappear (or become integrated by the brain) between 6 and 12 months.

You will see your baby's tongue extrusion reflex or response when you touch her tongue or lips. The touch stimulates forward tongue motion which is likely part of the suckle reflex or response. The tongue extrusion reflex may protect your baby from ingesting items for which she is not ready or are too large. Your baby begins to gain control over this reflex around 3 to 4 months, and it seems to disappear (or become integrated by the brain) between 12 and 18 months.

The swallowing reflex or response is triggered as saliva, liquid, and/or food move toward your baby's throat. A nutritive suck and swallow is approximately 1 per second with good suck-swallow-breathe synchrony (or rhythm). Most children gain control over swallowing around 18 months of age. It's an important reflex to retain throughout life. Without it, people need an alternate means of nutrition such as tube feeding.

Your baby's phasic bite reflex or response occurs when firm but gentle pressure is applied to her gums. This causes her to open and close her jaw in a rhythmic biting pattern (approximately 1 per second). The phasic bite reflex works the muscles which raise and lower the jaw, and these muscles are used in feeding and babbling. Your baby will begin to gain control of this reflex between 5 and 9 months, and it seems to disappear (or become integrated by the brain) between 9 and 12 months.

The transverse tongue reflex or response is stimulated by touch to either side of your baby's tongue. Her tongue moves toward the touch. This lateral or sideward tongue movement is ultimately used to place food for chewing and collect food for swallowing as your baby gains control over the reflex and as it become integrated by her brain. She begins to gain control of this reflex between 6 and 8 months, and it seems to disappear (or become integrated) between 9 and 24 months.

Your baby's gag reflex or response is stimulated by touch to the back ¾ of her tongue at birth. When stimulated, her mouth opens wide, her head may go back, her soft plate rises rapidly, and her voice box and diaphragm may rise. This reflex protects your baby from swallowing items that are too large. She begins to gain control of this reflex between 4 and 6 months. By 6 to 9 months her gag is usually found on back ⅓ of her tongue. The gag response typically continues throughout life on the back ¼ of the tongue in most people.

Hand-mouth reflexes are also present at birth. These are the palmomental, Babkin, and grasp responses. Hands and mouths work together as we see in feeding, eating, drinking, and speaking.

The palmomental reflex or response occurs when you touch the palm of your baby's hand. This results in the wrinkling or likely contraction of the mentalis muscles under the lower lip. The mentalis muscles evert (turn out) your baby's lower lip when she latches on the breast or bottle. These muscles are particularly active during breastfeeding. The palmomental reflex may be seen into adulthood in some people.

Your baby's Babkin reflex or response is stimulated by applying gentle pressure into the base of the palm in her hand. This results in your baby opening her mouth, closing her eyes, and moving her head forward, which likely helps prepare her to breastfeed. It may also be used in paced (baby-led) bottle-feeding. This reflex seems to disappear (or become integrated by the brain) around 3 to 4 months.

Your baby's grasp reflex or response is stimulated by gently pressing your baby's palm. It results in your baby grasping your finger. Her grasp tightens as she sucks, and she may also hold onto your clothing. This reflex seems to disappear (or become integrated by the brain) around 8 months.

The rooting, tongue extrusion, suckling, swallowing, palmomental, and Babkin reflexes seem related to sucking and early feeding. Rooting, suckling, and Babkin responses come under your baby's control between 1 and 4 months. The phasic bite, transverse tongue, gag, and grasp responses seem related to higher level feeding processes as these reflexes come under your baby's control between 4 and 9 months when your baby is learning open cup- and straw-drinking, spoon-feeding, taking bites of food, and chewing.

2

To Breastfeed and/or Bottle-Feed: That Is the Question

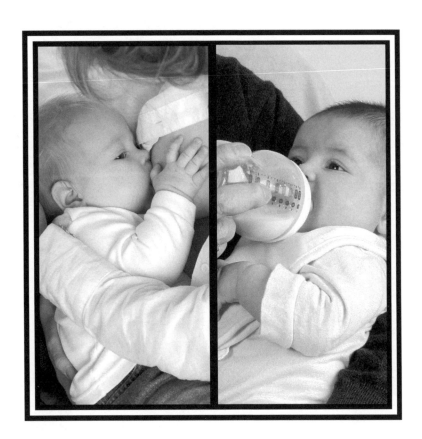

I would prefer all moms breastfeed their babies. However, I know this is not possible for some, so I don't want parents, particularly mothers, to feel guilty if they cannot breastfeed. I want you to know the benefits of breastfeeding whether you are breastfeeding and/or bottle-feeding. If you are bottle-feeding, you can help to counteract some of the negatives of bottle-feeding by understanding what breastfeeding does for a baby's mouth and airway development. This book contains both breastfeeding and bottle-feeding techniques to help you feed your baby in the best possible way whether you breastfeed, bottle-feed, or do a combination of both.

Breastfeeding and Bottle-Feeding Differences

While breastfeeding and bottle-feeding have some similarities, they are different processes. The differences are subtle for the untrained observer, but they exist. A mom often notices these as she prepares to return to work and transitions her baby to bottle-feeding, particularly after exclusively breastfeeding.

Breastfeeding and bottle-feeding have different movement characteristics and motor plans (sequences of movement programmed by the brain). As an adult example, think of the movement variations between driving a car with manual transmission versus one with an automatic transmission. Both allow you to drive the car, but they are different processes.

Here are some of the differences between breastfeeding and bottle-feeding.[98][99][100][101][102][103][104][105]

PROPERLY BREASTFEEDING BABIES	PROPERLY BOTTLE-FEEDING BABIES
Root to locate the mother's nipple.	Root if paced (baby-led) bottle-feeding is used.
Open the mouth fully for a wide, sustained latch on the breast.	Open the jaw only enough for the particular bottle nipple.
Extend the tongue over the lower lip to grasp the mother's breast.	Extend the tongue over the lower gum.
Draw the mother's nipple and breast deeply into the mouth, which helps maintain the broad "U" shaped roof of the mouth.	Use the lips and cheeks as a unit to latch onto the bottle.
Hold and cup the breast with the front of the tongue while the lips seal against the breast.	Cup the tongue if a rounded bottle nipple is used.
Lower the jaw and the front of the tongue together with little effort or cheek motion.	Have more cheek and lip movement than breastfed babies.
Use the mentalis (everts or turns out the lower lip for latch) and masseter (raises the jaw against gravity) muscles more than bottle-fed infants.	Use the mentalis and masseter muscles less than breastfed infants.

PROPERLY BREASTFEEDING BABIES continued	PROPERLY BOTTLE-FEEDING BABIES continued
Have more sucking movements with more and longer pauses than bottle-fed babies.	Have fewer sucking movements with fewer and shorter pauses than breastfed babies.
Move the back of the tongue in a wavelike manner essential for swallowing.	Move the back of the tongue downward to create a vacuum.[106]
Have a stable mouth with the tongue and lower jaw acting as the lower stabilizer, the sucking/fat pads (if present) acting as side stabilizers, and the relatively flat roof of the mouth acting as the top stabilizer.	Have a stable mouth with the tongue and lower jaw acting as the lower stabilizer, the cheeks and sucking pads (if present) acting as side stabilizers, and the roof of the mouth acting as the top stabilizer.
Have adequate pressure in the mouth, so fluid can move safely and efficiently into and through the mouth for swallowing.	Have adequate pressure in the mouth, so fluid can move safely and efficiently into and through the mouth for swallowing.
Have a good feeding rhythm.	Have a good feeding rhythm.

As you can see from the chart, a baby's mouth structures move in a more sophisticated manner during proper breastfeeding than during bottle-feeding. Breastfeeding also helps establish the sucking patterns we use throughout our lives in processes such as correct open cup-drinking, spoon-feeding, and straw-drinking. Proper breastfeeding supports suck-swallow-breathe coordination which assists the structures of the mouth and airway to work together as a "unified sensory-motor organ."[107] This leads to good mouth and airway development. Most full-term (40 weeks gestation) and close-to-term (37 to 39 weeks gestation) babies are born with the potential for breastfeeding, and

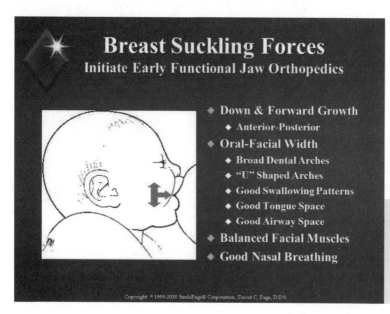

many premature babies can be aided in the development of breastfeeding. Breastfed babies root to locate the mom's nipple, and rooting leads directly into sucking. Many people don't realize the direct connection between rooting and sucking. Bottle-fed babies can root to suck if given the opportunity as in paced (baby-led) bottle-feeding.

Figure 2.1: *Dr. David C. Page, Sr. provides (with permission) a summary of mouth and airway development in a properly breastfed baby. Breastfeeding appears to be the only way to attain all of these characteristics beginning at birth.*

Breastfed babies open their mouths wide for the breast, using a full range of jaw motion for a wide and sustained latch. Bottle-fed babies open their jaws only wide enough for a particular bottle nipple using limited jaw range. Significant jaw growth and development occurs in the first year of life as the baby develops his many feeding skills. See the Feeding and Related Development Checklist: Birth to 24 Months in Chapter 1.

A breastfed baby extends his tongue over the lower lip to grasp the mom's breast and draw it deeply into his mouth. This helps maintain the broad "U" shape of the baby's mouth roof (upper palate), which is also the floor of the nasal area. Breastfed babies use the front of the tongue to hold and cup the mom's breast while their lips seal against the breast. The mentalis muscles (which assist lower lip movement) are active during breastfeeding. The breastfed baby lowers the jaw and front of the tongue together with ease. Little cheek movement is seen, and the back of the tongue moves in a wavelike manner for swallowing in breastfed babies.

In contrast, a bottle-fed baby extends his tongue over the lower gum, usually flares the lips as a unit to latch onto the bottle nipple, and may cup the tongue if drinking from a rounded bottle

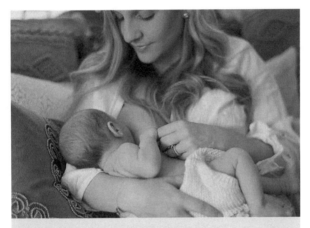

Photo 2.1: *Ali is breastfeeding Leo as a young infant. Breastfeeding is the best feeding method for good mouth and airway development while bottle-feeding is a medical way of feeding a baby. Photo provided with permission from Ali. Photographer: Nicky Alexandria Photography*

nipple. Tongue cupping is important for feeding, swallowing, and eventually speech. Bottle-fed babies use more cheek and lip movement and less mentalis and masseter movement than breastfed infants. Exclusively breastfed babies have different sucking patterns than bottle-fed babies. Bottle-fed babies have fewer sucking movements with fewer and shorter pauses than babies who are solely breastfed.[108]

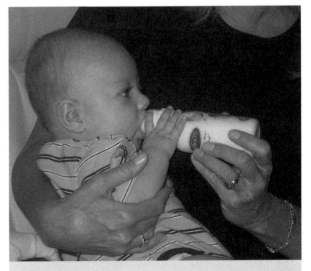

Photo 2.2: *Paced (baby led) bottle-feeding is used with Anthony at 4 months. He has a nice hand-mouth connection. You can see how his lips and cheeks are working as a unit. As you know, bottle-feeding is a different process than breastfeeding.*

Therefore, bottle-fed infants seem to move their mouth structures as units, while properly breastfed babies seem to move these structures in an independent but unified manner. The more sophisticated movements of breastfeeding relative to bottle feeding also appear to support later-developing feeding skills such as appropriate open cup- and straw-drinking, chewing, etc.[109]

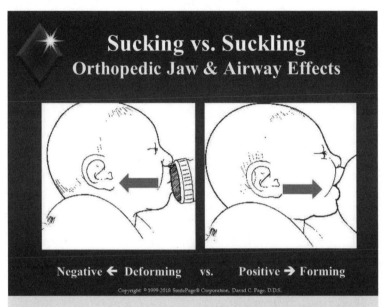

Figure 2.2: *Dr. David C. Page, Sr. provides (with permission) a visual summary of the negative impact of bottle-feeding vs. the positive impact of breastfeeding on jaw and airway development. Bottle-fed babies are subject to unnatural forces that pull the jaw backward, while breastfed babies' jaws can grow forward secondary to the balanced and natural pressures involved in breastfeeding.*

Health and Development Benefits of Breastfeeding versus Bottle-Feeding

Breastfeeding has fortunately made a comeback as the preferred infant feeding method for many reasons. Most importantly, breastfeeding is biologically normal. It provides the mom and baby with significant health and development benefits. Breastfeeding is supported by the World Health Organization (WHO), the American Academy of Pediatrics (AAP), and many other groups around the world. In fact, an article in the AAP journal (2010) revealed breastfeeding is medically cost effective and saves baby's lives.[110] Bottle-feeding began as a compensatory medical process for children who could not breastfeed. It became increasingly prevalent as countries were industrialized and mothers went to work. As you discovered in the previous section of this chapter, bottle-feeding is a different and apparently less sophisticated process than breastfeeding.

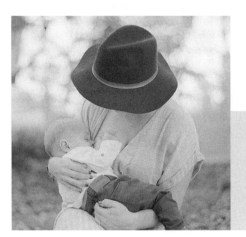

Photo 2.3: *Ali is breastfeeding Leo at 6 months. Breastfed children have a lower incidence of ear and respiratory problems, insulin-dependent diabetes and obesity, reflux and gastrointestinal problems, and sudden infant death syndrome. They also tend to have better immune systems, mouth and airway growth, and speech development than bottle-fed babies. Photo provided with permission from Ali. Photographer: Nicky Alexandria Photography*

A breastfeeding mom feeds her baby on alternate breasts, providing equal exercise and stimulation to both sides of her baby's face, head, and body.[111] Parents who bottle-feed can use paced (baby-led) bottle-feeding and alternate the sides on which they feed their baby, but this will not compensate for the other exercise benefits of breastfeeding. As previously mentioned, the rooting reflex leads the breastfed baby into sucking. Bottle-fed babies usually don't have the opportunity to root unless paced (baby-led) bottle-feeding is used, so they miss the preparation rooting appears to supply for sucking.

When a baby breastfeeds properly, the breast is drawn deeply into the infant's mouth. This helps maintain the broad "U" shape of the mouth's roof (palate), which is also the floor of the nasal area. No bottle nipple (or pacifier) can do this. The wide "U" shape of the upper palate is also maintained by the baby keeping the tongue against the palate when the mouth is closed at rest. On the other hand, bottle-fed babies (particularly those who concurrently use a pacifier) often develop high, narrow palates and resulting small nasal areas, as well as ear problems.[112] [113] This is likely related to unnatural and compensatory processes and forces involved in bottle-feeding. See Breastfeeding and Bottle-Feeding Differences in the previous section of this chapter. Some breastfed babies may also develop high, narrow palates and small nasal areas if they have tongue ties or are breastfeeding incorrectly.

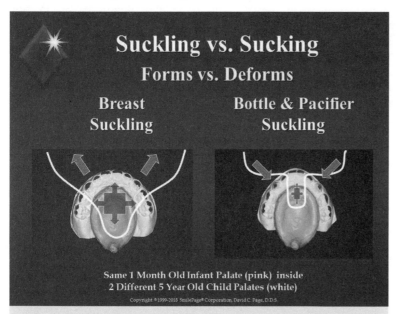

Figure 2.3: *Dr. David C. Page, Sr. provides (with permission) the comparison of upper palate development (mouth roof) in babies and children who breastfeed vs. those who bottle-feed. You can see the narrowing of the palate in the bottle-fed baby which also negatively impacts overall mouth development as well as the nasal and sinus areas (airway).*

A high, narrow palate and resulting small nasal area can make nasal breathing difficult, forcing the baby to mouth-breathe. Persistent mouth-breathing is extremely unhealthy.[114] [115] [116] [117] [118] Children who mouth-breathe on a regular basis are not filtering the air through the nasal structures and do not breath as deeply as children who nose-breathe. Continual mouth-breathing has been connected with enlarged tonsils and adenoids, allergies, asthma, ear problems, sinus problems, reflux, stress, obstructive sleep disorders, blood pressure concerns, heart problems, and attention problems.

Bottle-fed infants are generally sicker than successfully breastfed infants.[119] This makes sense if you think about a high, narrow palate making the nasal and sinus areas small and difficult to clear, likely forcing the baby to mouth-breathe. Breastfed babies have fewer allergies, ear, nasal, and sinus problems,[120] other respiratory infections,[121] insulin-dependent diabetes,[122] as well as less reflux and other gastrointestinal problems.[123] They are also less likely to be overweight or to die from Sudden Infant Death Syndrome (SIDS).[124 125 126] Properly breastfed babies have better immune systems, as well as better mouth and airway development than those who bottle-feed. Face, jaw, dental arch, palate, tooth, and speech development is better in breastfed than bottle-fed infants.[127 128 129 130 131]

Bottle-feeding can result in underdeveloped jaws, narrowing of the mouth and facial structures, and subsequent orthodontic problems.[132] In fact, recent research continues to indicate bottle-feeding negatively impacts the growth and development of the top and bottom jaws, interfering with primary tooth development and ultimately leading to problems with dental occlusion.[133 134 135 136 137] These difficulties are likely related to the different sucking patterns used in bottle-feeding versus breastfeeding. The sucking patterns used in bottle-feeding are also similar to detrimental patterns used during pacifier; incorrect straw, spouted-cup, and pouch food use; as well as thumb, finger, and blanket sucking.

According to Dr. David C. Page, Sr. considered a pioneer in functional jaw orthopedics, breastfeeding is the best way to ensure proper jaw growth. The jaw is the keystone for the development of other structures around it such as the nasal area, lips, cheeks, and tongue. It's "the gateway to the human airway."[138] Dr. Page, Sr. says the movements of breastfeeding assist jaw growth, which occurs rapidly during the first year of life. If the jaw is not doing what it needs to do, the lips and tongue cannot do what they need to do. It is also true that if the tongue is not doing what it needs to do, the jaw may not grow properly. This is often the case with tongue tie. Dr. Page, Sr. recommends breastfeeding over bottle-feeding whenever possible. He says "bottle, pacifier,

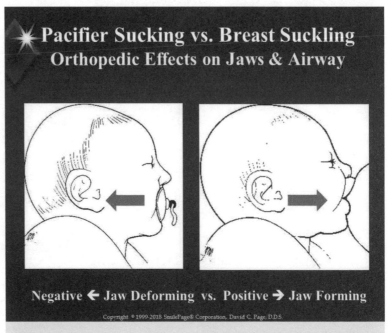

Figure 2.4: *Dr. David C. Page, Sr. provides (with permission) a visual summary of the negative impact of pacifier use vs. the positive impact of breastfeeding on jaw and airway development. Pacifier, spouted cup, and pouch food use, as well as long-term thumb and finger sucking pull the jaw backward, while breastfeeding assists with positive forward jaw growth secondary to the balanced and natural pressures involved in breastfeeding.*

and digit sucking create backward destructive forces on both upper and lower jaws."[139] These forces can narrow the dental arches and palate, ultimately causing malocclusion.[140 141 142 143 144 145 146] Some malocclusions include over-bite, over-jet, under-bite, cross-bite,[147] open bite, crooked or crowded teeth, and other jaw problems.

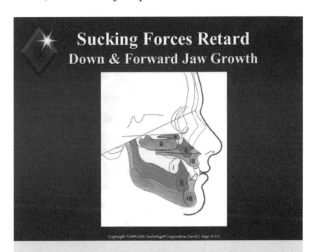

Figure 2.5: *Dr. David C. Page, Sr. provides (with permission) a view of good, balanced down and forward jaw growth. This diagram shows how the first year of life is a most rapid period of jaw growth. The backward sucking forces of bottle, pacifier, spouted cup, and pouch food use put unnatural backward forces on the jaw.*

Dr. Ashley Montagu, a social scientist, presented significant research on breastfeeding from many different fields of study and cultures in the book *Touching: The Human Significance of the Skin*.[148] Dr. Montagu discussed one study of 173 children followed from birth to 10 years of age. Babies who were breastfed had 4 times fewer respiratory infections, 20 times fewer bouts of diarrhea, 22 times fewer infections of other kinds, 8 times fewer cases of eczema, 20 times fewer cases of asthma, and 27 times fewer cases hay fever.[149] Another study of 383 children found bottle-fed

children were nutritionally poorer, more susceptible to childhood diseases, and slower to learn walking and talking than breastfed children.[150] Both Drs. Page, Sr. and Montagu comment on the research suggesting higher intelligence and physical health in breastfed children.[151 152]

The superior physical health of breastfed children seems related to good airway development and qualities found in breast milk compared to formula. Breastfeeding supports proper airway development. The airway consists of your baby's nose, throat, windpipe, and voice box leading to the lungs. Upper airway development is dependent upon appropriate jaw and face growth.[153] Airway obstruction can cause

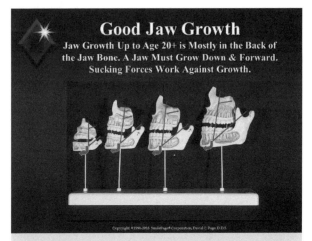

Figure 2.6: *Dr. David C. Page, Sr. provides (with permission) what good, balanced down and forward jaw growth should be over time as a child grows. Appropriate breastfeeding, open cup- and straw-use, taking bites of food and chewing, as well as intentional, supervised tummy or belly time, creeping, and crawling assist with this process. However, sucking on bottles, pacifiers, spouted cups, and pouch foods places upward and backward forces on the jaws and eventually the teeth. This often results in significant mouth and airway problems.*

unhealthy, chronic mouth-breathing, as well as changes in face and jaw development.[154] As previously mentioned, there is a connection between airway obstruction, allergies, asthma, ear problems, nasal and sinus problems, reflux, and stress.[155] Obstructive sleep disorders, blood pressure concerns, and heart problems can be added to this list.[156][157] Proper airway development is essential for a child's health.

Pediatric obstructive sleep apnea is now a significant concern. Dr. Christian Guilleminault and Dr. Yu-Shu Huang (pediatric sleep medicine specialists) have written extensively on this topic.[158][159][160] The journal *Pediatrics: Official Journal of the American Academy of Pediatrics* also contains a number of articles on childhood obstructive sleep apnea, such as those by Dr. Karen Bonuck and her colleagues.[161][162][163] Proper breastfeeding and the release of tethered oral tissues (such as tongue tie) seem to be the best possible way to maintain a well-developing upper airway in young infants. The need for many procedures in older babies and children (such as tonsil and adenoid removal, as well as significant orthodontic work) may be avoided or reduced through the use of correct breastfeeding practices, tethered oral tissue releases, proper feeding techniques, and appropriate mouth development activities.

There are ways to treat pediatric obstructive sleep apnea as a child ages, but this is beyond the scope of this book. These processes usually require the use of specific oral appliances and surgeries (palatal expanders, braces, tonsillectomy, adenoidectomy, and other procedures).[164][165][166] There are now teams of professionals including otolaryngologists (ear, nose, and throat doctors: ENTs), dentists, orthodontists, cranial osteopaths, orofacial myofunctional therapists, and others who treat pediatric obstructive sleep apnea.[167] For example, Dr. Barry Raphael (integrative orthodontist) has a treatment and educational setting where a variety of professionals come together to treat and learn about the many aspects of mouth and airway structure and function.

Dr. David Ingram (pediatrician and sleep physician) wrote the book *Sleep Apnea in Children: A Handbook for Families* (2018).[168] Dr. Michael Gelb (integrative dentist) and Dr. Howard Hindin (integrative dentist) wrote the book *Gasp! Airway Health—The Hidden Path to Wellness* (2016). This book is an easy-to-read resource on airway and related health problems across the life span.[169] Dr. David C. Page, Sr. (functional jaw orthopedist and integrative dentist) wrote a parent- and professional-friendly book on the importance of adequate jaw development for good health entitled *Your Jaws – Your Life* (2014).[170]

The World Health Organization recommends exclusive breastfeeding during the first 6 months of life for optimum infant health, growth, and development. Breastfeeding may continue until age 2 years or beyond in some cases. Nutritious, appropriate, and complementary foods are introduced at age 6 months.[171][172] These guidelines are similar to recommendations from the American Academy of Pediatrics. However, at times pediatricians may recommend feeding complementary foods to specific children prior to 6 months in developed countries with a safe food supply. Discuss this with your child's pediatrician.

As you can see, there is a significant amount of research to support the value of breastfeeding for good and appropriate mouth and airway development. However, if you need to bottle-feed your baby, we will discuss some of the best possible methods in Chapter 3.

Why Are So Many Moms Having Difficulty Breastfeeding?

Breastfeeding difficulties are often related to problems within the baby's mouth such as thin or non-existent sucking pads, tethered oral tissues (such as tongue and lip ties), and/or mild jaw weakness. Yet, many moms erroneously think the problem is milk supply, inverted nipples, or another problem the mom is having. However, it is often the baby who has a difference in mouth structure and function causing the difficulty.

Breastfeeding difficulties may also be related to other factors. We live in a different world than our hunting and gathering predecessors. Moms often work in sedentary jobs, may not sleep well, and may not breathe properly. This can affect a mom's overall health and a baby's oxygen supply. Our diets are not local and seasonal, which may impact both the mom's and the baby's nutrition. Baby deliveries are mostly medicalized with processes like epidurals and birthing on the back. Many babies are not given the opportunity to do the breast crawl, and umbilical cords are usually cut quickly.[173][174][175][176] The breast crawl allows the baby to make his way to the breast and latch after birth. Additionally, the baby was attached to the umbilical cord for many months to supply him with oxygen and nutrients, yet the cord is often cut very quickly. I often wonder how this affects the baby.[177]

Breastfeeding moms usually have the advantage of working with International Board-Certified Lactation Consultants (IBCLCs). If you are planning to breastfeed, find an IBCLC with whom you feel comfortable before giving birth, if possible. Many hospitals have these specialists available to mothers at birth. Moms need support early and often if they have any difficulties with breastfeeding.

IBCLCs often work with other specially trained professionals when complex breastfeeding concerns arise. These professionals may be in the fields of speech-language pathology, orofacial myology, dentistry, otolaryngology, cranial osteopathy, chiropractic, occupational therapy, physical therapy, etc. IBCLCs also have access to important tools and techniques for the best breastfeeding results and can help parents supplement their children with other feeding methods (such as syringes, open cups, a supplemental feeding system, nipple shields, bottle-feeding, etc.) until the mom and baby can work through difficulties with breastfeeding.

Babies who bottle-feed can also receive benefits from drinking pumped breast milk. Breast milk is a complete food. It contains a variety of tastes and good nutrition as long as Mom has a well-rounded, healthy diet. It also contains natural antibodies.[178][179][180] This is one reason babies who drink breast milk have fewer allergy, ear, nasal, and sinus problems; less reflux and gastrointestinal problems; and better immune systems. Additionally, pumped breast milk tends to agree with the baby's digestive system better than most formulas which cannot replicate the value provided by breast milk.

The International Lactation Consultant Association (ILCA) has wonderful breastfeeding information on their site in addition to a directory for finding an International Board-Certified Lactation Consultant (IBCLC). The United States Lactation Association also offers good resources and a directory in the USA. Kellymom and the La Leche League International are other excellent, literature-based resources for breastfeeding. Additionally, the book *Supporting Sucking Skills in Breastfeeding Infants* (2017) by Catherine Watson Genna and others is an evidence-based resource about how to have successful breastfeeding when there are sucking problems.[181]

In my practice, I see many moms and babies who have difficulty breastfeeding. They are referred by knowledgeable IBCLCs, pediatric dentists, and physicians who want to know why breastfeeding is failing. Many moms use nipple shields for latch, mouth, upper airway, and nipple problems.[182] While nipple shields can be very helpful for these reasons, the baby basically sucks from a nipple shield in the same way as a bottle nipple. When these babies are placed at the breast (without a nipple shield), they often have very shallow and weak latches initially. So, it's important to work with an IBCLC on this process.

Many babies with breastfeeding difficulties have tongue and/or lip ties (as well as other issues such as thin or missing sucking pads and mild jaw weakness). It would be ideal if every baby was screened for tethered oral tissues and had ties released at birth. This practice is already in place in Brazil. IBCLCs could then work with moms and babies on proper breastfeeding without tongue and lip restrictions. However, many babies and children have the release(s) well after birth. With these children, I prefer to work with parents and babies, as well as their IBCLC before and after the release to teach pre-release work and help prepare the parents for essential post-release work. The IBCLC is my partner in this process and is usually the person who works frequently and consistently with the parents and baby until the baby is feeding well.

If a baby's restriction has been released by laser and the parents have done the required stretches for wound care, I usually work with the baby and parents on age-appropriate jaw, tongue, lip, and cheek movements for feeding. If the stretches have not been done, the baby may need another revision because the wound may have developed scar tissue. If the baby has been released by a scalpel or scissors with sutures, I usually work on age-appropriate jaw, tongue, lip, and cheek movements for feeding with the baby and parents as soon as the surgeon gives permission for these activities to begin (usually within days of the procedure). See section on Tongue, Lip, and Buccal Restrictions in this chapter. As you know, I prefer to work along with an IBCLC and other appropriate professionals during the process. A team approach is best, and the parents and baby are part of the team.

The other problem I frequently encounter with babies who have breastfeeding difficulties is missing or limited sucking pads. When a baby does not have appropriate sucking pads, the cheek areas collapse and there is too much room in the baby's mouth to attain adequate pressure for sucking. The breastfeeding mom usually needs to carefully apply cheek support in the form of the *dancer hand position or a modified dancer hold*, so the baby can attain the intraoral pressure needed to suck, swallow, and breathe efficiently and effectively. We will discuss these hand positions in Chapter 3.

Sucking (fat) pads develop toward the end of pregnancy when the fat is developing on the rest of the baby's body, so premature babies will not have them and close-to-term babies (37 to 39 weeks gestation) may have thin ones. Sucking pads do not develop after birth. Some full-term babies (40 weeks gestation) may also be born with thin or missing sucking pads. Sucking pads are essential for mouth stability during breastfeeding. Therefore, compensatory methods are needed when they are missing or thin.

So, what is going on, and why are so many problems occurring? Pediatric dentist Kevin Boyd studies and discusses changes in human mouth development that seem related to changes in inherited genes (epigenetics).[183] [184] Many of these changes appear related to feeding practices used over the generations such as the introduction of medical bottle-feeding and eating soft, convenience foods. Pouch foods and the ground meat found in chicken nuggets are examples of soft, convenience foods. Integrative dentist Dr. Steven Lin also discusses these issues and recommends a diet for reversing the problem in his book *The Dental Diet: The Surprising Link Between Your Teeth, Real Food, and Life-Changing Natural Health* (2018).[185] Improper and inappropriate feeding and eating practices seem to be changing the human species over time. Therefore, underdeveloped jaws, tongue and lip ties, as well as limited or missing sucking pads may be related to changes in the ways we have been eating, drinking, and feeding over several generations.

Additionally, the daily positioning we now use with babies likely impacts the changes we are seeing in overall body development. Babies often spend very little time on their tummies or sides and spend an inordinate amount of time on their backs. They seem to go from *required sleeping on the back* to a variety of types of containers (such as car seats, swings, and baby seats). Therefore, many

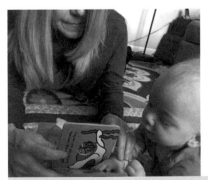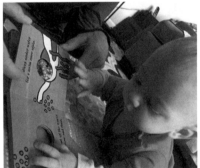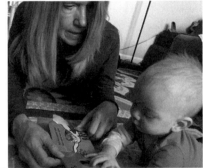

Photo 2.4: *Cannon (6.5 months) and Diane look at books together in supervised, intentional belly time. It's also a great position for adults.*

babies are placed into positions where gravity cannot help with full body development (such as the advancement of core or postural control and forward jaw growth). In fact, the continuous placement of babies on their backs and/or in containers is likely contributing to the delays many therapists, pediatricians, and parents now see in gross and fine motor skill progression. This information is detailed in the Intentional, Supervised Tummy/Belly Time to Creeping/Crawling Checklist: A Likely Fundamental Missing Developmental Link (Birth to 7 Months) in Chapter 1.

Belly time, side-lying, and other body positions (supervised and intentional beginning at birth); as well as rolling, creeping, and crawling are fundamental for good overall body development. These activities involve front-to-back, side-to-side, diagonal, and rotational body movements. If these movements don't occur in the body, they are unlikely to occur in the mouth (an area of fine motor function). This probably contributes to poor jaw development, as well as late tooth eruption, feeding, speaking, and other skills. See the Crucial Developmental Checklists in Chapter 1.

Tongue, Lip, and Buccal Restrictions

While most people have tongue and lip frenums (tissues attaching the tongue to floor of the mouth and the lips to the gums), some children are born with significant restrictions in these tissues that inhibit or limit typical mouth movement. These are referred to as *frenum restrictions*, *ties*, or *tethered oral tissues*. Restrictions result in tightness that keeps a structure or structures from moving and functioning properly. They can significantly limit jaw, tongue, lip, and cheek movements which are functions needed for effective and efficient feeding, as well as overall mouth and airway development.[186]

Ideally, all babies should be screened for tongue, lip, and buccal (cheek) ties at birth. However, this is not routinely done. These restrictions often occur in utero during early mouth development.[187] They are believed to result from remaining stretch-resistant tissues (type 1 collagen) which have not resorbed into the body during gestation in a process called apoptosis or programmed cell death. Therefore, these types of restrictions resist stretching and require surgery to be released.[188][189] They can also be inherited, and boys seem more impacted than girls.[190][191][192]

Babies suckle and suck in utero, so those with significant tongue and lip ties are born using maladaptive, compensatory sucking movements. These compensatory movements can cause significant deviations in mouth and face structures and functions as the baby grows, ultimately resulting in the need for orthodontic and/or other treatments. In breastfeeding, restrictions (such as tongue tie) may be indicated by latching difficulties, nipple problems (misshapen, sore, painful, cracked, or bleeding nipples), plugged milk ducts, gastrointestinal issues (gastroesophageal reflux, gassiness, etc.), or difficulty calming the baby. However, there may be other problems causing or contributing to these issues—such as limited sucking pads or subtle muscle function problems (often mild jaw weakness). If you think your child has a tongue or lip tie, see a qualified professional who regularly diagnoses and treats these problems.

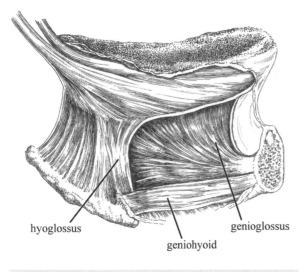

hyoglossus

geniohyoid

genioglossus

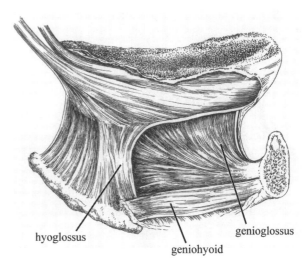

hyoglossus

geniohyoid

genioglossus

*"With **anterior tongue tie** (classic tongue tie), the shortened frenulum attaches to the tip (or several millimeters from the tip) of the tongue and attaches to the mandible. These more obvious cases of tongue tie can limit elevation, retroflexion, lateralization and protrusion."*

Figure 2.7: *Drawings and quotes provided by Bobak Ghaheri, MD, ENT, (drghaheri.com) with his permission.*

*"**Posterior tongue tie** is present when restriction of the middle tongue exists while the anterior tongue is mobile. There is absence of a significant visible frenulum, but the genioglossus muscle is restricted by abnormal collagenous fascial attachments. This type of restriction is most noticeable with elevation and retroflexion. Often, children with posterior tongue tie may seemingly protrude the tongue well, but further inspection indicates that the band under the tongue forces the tongue to curl down in an arc."*

There are different types of tongue ties: anterior (front), posterior (back), mucosal, or submucosal (hidden). As previously mentioned, these can keep the tongue from moving properly during breast-feeding[193] and bottle-feeding. They can also prevent typical mouth function for eating, drinking, and speaking as the child ages. A tongue tie can result in a high, narrow roof of the mouth. The tongue

Photo 2.5: *Photos and descriptions provided with permission by Dr. Larry Kotlow, pediatric dentist (www.kidsteeth.com). Dr. Kotlow is the author of* SOS 4 TOTS: Tethered Oral Tissues, Tongue-Ties & Lip-Ties *(2016).*

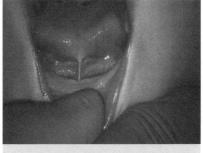

Class IV Anterior Tongue Tie

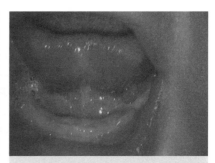

Class II Posterior Tongue Tie

is meant to rest in the upper palate (mouth roof) to help maintain its broad "U" shape. The roof of the mouth is the floor of the nasal area. If the upper palate becomes high and narrow, the nasal area usually becomes small and difficult to clear which may result in unhealthy mouth-breathing.

Chronic open mouth-breathing is not normal and can contribute to significant health problems if left untreated. Children who mouth-breathe often have enlarged tonsils and/or adenoids, allergies, increased respiratory illness, problems with tooth eruption and decay, heart problems, low-resting tongue position, tongue thrust or abnormal oral swallow, as well as sleep-disordered breathing.[194][195][196][197][198] Nose-breathing is normal and natural for human beings. Nasal-breathing filters debris and pathogens from the air that can cause illness. It also warms the air and encourages deep breathing needed for body movement, blood oxygenation, good metabolism, and overall health. Additionally, nose-breathing can reduce stress.

While little research is available on lip and cheek ties, a significant lip tie may impact breastfeeding, bottle-feeding, eating, drinking, dental development, and speaking. In particular, a substantial restriction of tissue between the upper lip and gum can keep a baby from obtaining an appropriate lip latch on the breast or bottle.

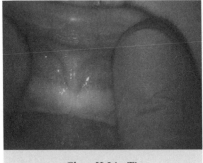

Class II Lip Tie

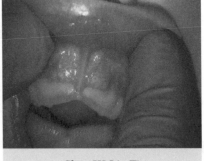

Class III Lip Tie

Photo 2.6: *Photos and descriptions provided with permission by Dr. Larry Kotlow, pediatric dentist (www.kidsteeth.com). Dr. Kotlow is the author of* SOS 4 TOTS: Tethered Oral Tissues, Tongue-Ties & Lip-Ties *(2016).*

Cheek (buccal) restrictions can limit lip and cheek movement as cheeks help to activate lips. Large buccal ties may interfere with oral hygiene as the child gets older, but these are often left unrevised unless the ties significantly impact cheek movement or pull the gums away from the teeth. In my experience, I have seen tongue and lip ties occurring together. So, if one area is restricted, it's important to check for other restrictions. Some restrictions (those *not caused* by type 1 collagen) may be resolved through the use of appropriate feeding and facilitation techniques (such as massage, stretching, and exercise). These restrictions are likely caused by improper use of the tongue muscles.

Babies with significant restrictions, usually resulting from remaining stretch-resistant tissues that limit normal mouth function, require surgical intervention using a laser, scalpel, or another appropriate instrument as designated by the treating provider. A properly trained dentist, oral surgeon, otolaryngologist (ear, nose, and throat doctor: ENT), pediatrician, or other physician typically completes the surgery. Two procedures most widely used to release tethered oral tissues are *frenotomy* (separating tissue) and *frenectomy* (removing some tissue).[199] These can be simple outpatient procedures with minimal pain depending on the child and the skill of the surgeon. Look for providers in your area with the proper training, experience, and follow-up care.

Additionally, it's important to choose the procedure that is right for you and your child. While a laser procedure may be a good procedure for a baby or child who will tolerate the required stretches during aftercare or wound care, a scalpel or scissor procedure with sutures may work well for a child who may not allow the stretches or is deemed better suited for this procedure by your surgeon. Some doctors, such as Dr. Soroush Zaghi, perform functional *frenuloplasty* (a form of frenectomy involving blunt and sharp dissection for complete release of tethered oral tissues with repair of the overlying mucosa). This procedure is performed by scalpel or scissors with some form of anesthesia (local or general) depending on the age and cooperation of the child. The wound heals by primary intention because the wound edges are brought together by sutures. Within days of this procedure, the child usually begins age-appropriate oral activities (feeding, motor speech, and/or oral sensory-motor activities) with guidance from an appropriately trained therapist once the physician gives permission for treatment.

Other doctors use a laser to release tethered oral tissues. This process heals by secondary intention where the edges of the wound are not brought together for healing. So, specific daily stretches are required for a period of time to help the mouth heal properly. Some laser surgery can be done without anesthesia.

The type of procedure chosen is usually dependent on the parent, child, and provider. Here are just a few websites, so you can explore some of the differences:

PROFESSIONAL	WEBSITE
Dr. Rajeev Agarwal, Pediatrician	www.agavepediatrics.com
Dr. Bobak (Bobby) Ghaheri, Otolaryngologist	www.drghaheri.com
Dr. Marjan Jones, Integrative Dentist	www.enhancedentistry.com.au
Dr. Lawrence (Larry) Kotlow, Pediatric Dentist	www.kiddsteeth.com
Dr. Shahrzad (Sherry) Sami, Pediatric Dentist and Orthodontist	www.happykidsdentalplanet.com
Dr. Soroush Zaghi, Sleep Surgeon Sanda Valcu-Pinkerton, Myofunctional Therapist	www.zaghimd.com www.thebreatheinstitute.com www.myofunctionaltherapyla.com

In my practice, I like to provide both before- and after-care for these surgical procedures unless the tissues are released at birth; then, after-care is in order. Before the procedure, I like to evaluate and facilitate as much range of motion in the structures as possible. The after-care consists of supporting parents in tongue lifts (with laser surgery) and teaching the child how to move the jaw, tongue, lips, and cheeks in a typical manner for eating, drinking, and speaking (once the surgeon agrees we can work on these processes). Appropriate feeding, eating, and drinking activities are covered in this book, but the other activities and information can be found in *Nobody Every Told Me (or My Mother) That! Everything from Bottles and Breathing to Healthy Speech Development* by Diane Bahr (Chapters 4, 5, 7, and 8).

This process is similar to the aftercare provided for most surgeries, where body parts learn to move properly through rehabilitation and daily home practice. A tethered oral tissue release is a relatively simple procedure, and after-care exercises and stretches can be part of a child's daily routine. They usually only take minutes to do as part of oral hygiene, feeding, and play. Parents need to seek well-trained professionals to guide them in appropriate before- and after-care. In my opinion, a team approach is best. The team often includes the surgeon, an oral sensory-motor therapist (someone who works specifically with feeding and mouth function), a qualified pediatric body worker (someone who works with the child's entire body), the parents, the baby, and others as needed.

IBCLCs, feeding therapists, and orofacial myofunctional therapists work with mouth function. Feeding therapists are usually speech-language pathologists or occupational therapists who have significant experience with feeding. Orofacial myofunctional therapists are speech-language pathologists or dental professionals who are specially trained in attaining correct resting tongue position (in the roof of the mouth), a mature oral phase swallowing pattern, and many other related processes. The *oral phase* of the swallow is the part that happens in the mouth.

Cranial osteopaths, physical therapists, craniosacral therapists, massage therapists, and others are trained in body work. I personally have training in full-body massage, craniosacral treatment, myofascial release, and other modalities. I am also a certified infant massage instructor. However, I send the babies and children with whom I work to a professional who specializes in body work, so I can focus on the child's feeding, eating, drinking, and/or speech. As we discussed early in the book, the whole body works together. If the child's body is not moving and functioning properly, then it is difficult for the mouth to move and function well.

Here some other resources on tethered oral tissues:

- *Color Atlas of Infant Tongue-Tie and Lip-Tie Laser Frenectomy* by Robert Convissar, Alison Hazelbaker, Martin Kaplan, and Peter Vitruk [200]

- *Demystify the Tongue Tie: Methods to Confidently Analyze and Treat A Tethered Tongue* by Char Boshart [201]

- *Functional Assessment and Remediation of Tethered Oral Tissues* by Robyn Merkel-Walsh and Lori L. Overland [202]

- *Please Release Me: The Tethered Oral Tissue (TOT) Puzzle* by Patricia Pine [203]

- *SOS 4 TOTS: Tethered Oral Tissues, Tongue-Ties & Lip Ties* by Lawrence A. Kotlow [204]

- *Supporting Sucking Skills in Breastfeeding Infants* (Third ed.) by Catherine Watson Genna and other authors [205]

- *Tongue Tie: Breastfeeding and Beyond. A Parents' Guide to Diagnosis, Division and Aftercare* by Catherine Horsfall [206]

- *Tongue Tie—from Confusion to Clarity: A Guide to the Diagnosis and Treatment of Ankyloglossia* by Carmen Fernando [207]

- *Tongue-Tie: Morphogenesis, Impact, Assessment and Treatment* by Alison Hazelbaker [208]

3

Good Breastfeeding and Bottle-Feeding Practices and What to Do If Problems Arise

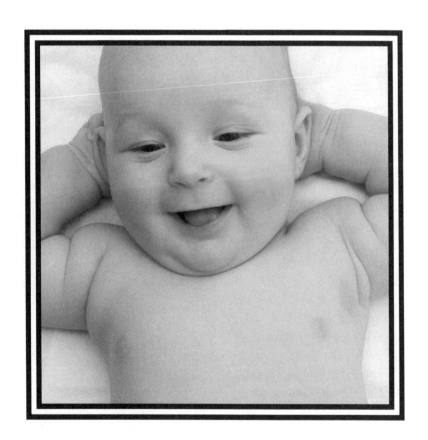

The Best Positioning for Feeding Your Baby and Why

Positioning can also affect your baby's ability to feed properly. Whether you have chosen to breastfeed and/or bottle-feed, see if you can follow these guidelines to find an optimal feeding position for you and your baby.

During breastfeeding:

1. Keep your baby's head in alignment with his body (head, neck, and body in a straight line). Your lactation consultant (preferably an IBCLC) may teach you to have your baby latch by leading with the chin. This can help your baby open the mouth wide, so the breast can be drawn deeply into his or her mouth. Once your baby is latched, his nose may be close to your breast (depending on the positioning you use). This allows proper extension in your baby's neck without hyperextension (head and neck too far back). A breastfed baby should maintain a wide, sustained latch.

2. Do not allow your baby's head and neck to extend too far backward. Head and neck hyperextension can cause some irregular patterns to occur in your baby's mouth. These patterns include excessive jaw movement (such as chomping), too much tongue protrusion, tongue humping or bunching (never normal), and biting down for stability (ouch for the breastfeeding mom).

3. Work with your lactation consultant (preferably an IBCLC) on the ideal breastfeeding position(s) for you and your baby. A directory of board-certified lactation consultants is available at www.ilca.org. As you know, I recommend you work with an International Board-Certified Lactation Consultant (IBCLC).

I personally like the laid-back position, which is a natural breastfeeding position. It's the position your baby would assume if he did the breast crawl at birth. In this position, you are reclined at a comfortable angle (perhaps 45+ degrees), and your baby is lying belly-to-belly with you. His head and feet are positioned with the same orientation as your head and feet (head up and feet down). His mouth is at your breast, and his jaw is being guided forward by gravity as he opens his mouth wide to latch onto your breast. A breastfed baby should maintain a wide, sustained latch. Most babies are born with retruded, or retrognathic, lower jaws, which appear small and pulled back. In the laid-back breastfeeding position, your baby

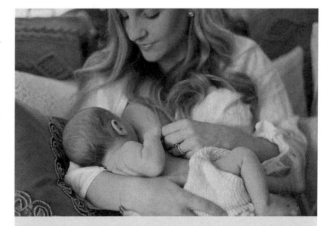

Photo 3.1: *Ali is breastfeeding Leo in a beautiful cradle position. Leo's body is nicely aligned. Ali is well-supported and a bit reclined. She looks very relaxed. Photo provided with permission from Ali. Photographer: Nicky Alexandria Photography*

has control of the milk coming from your breast rather than gravity controlling your milk flow, and he can make eye contact with you.

Suzanne Colson and her colleagues have written a number of articles about breastfeeding positioning.[209][210][211] The articles discuss research and include photos of appropriate breastfeeding positions. Colson and her colleagues demonstrate newborns may naturally be abdominal (belly) feeders, with antigravity reflexes assisting the wide, sustained latch. This supports the use of the laid-back breastfeeding position which helps your baby's jaw grow forward (vital for appropriate jaw development).

I also find the cradle hold to be a good position if a baby has thin or missing sucking pads, as the mom can express some breast milk to get the baby started or continue with feeding. Mom can also use a dancer or modified dancer hold in this position to give the baby carefully applied cheek support to compensate for thin or missing sucking pads which do not develop after birth. We will discuss carefully applied cheek support in a later section of this chapter.[212][213][214][215][216][217][218][219][220]

Some moms initially breastfeed in side-lying if the baby has a weak latch. This is where you rest on your side with your head on an appropriate, comfortable pillow and your baby's head may rest on your lower arm or a properly folded towel. Then the hand of your upper arm can assist with expressing milk and providing carefully applied cheek support if needed. Side-lying removes some of the effects of gravity. It also allows the mom to express milk to help the baby suck and use a dancer or modified dancer hand position (discussed later in this chapter) if the baby has missing or thin sucking pads. Once the mom and baby have a rhythm in this position, the mom can move upright into a laid-back breastfeeding position from side-lying. Other holds, such as the cross-cradle hold and the football hold, can likewise be very effective. You can breastfeed in any position that works for you and your baby. Your lactation consultant (preferably an IBCLC) will help you find a good position. This may even mean you feed your baby on one breast more than the other based on your IBCLC's recommendations.

If your baby is breastfeeding properly, it's unlikely fluid will enter his Eustachian tubes because the pressures within the mouth and nasopharynx are equalized. Breast milk is living tissue, and macrophage cell activity destroys most bacteria if breast milk should enter the Eustachian tubes.[221] Macrophage cells are the most numerous cells in breast milk. They appear to have antibacterial characteristics to assist the baby in the development of a healthy immune system.[222][223][224][225] We will discuss Eustachian tubes in the next section.

During bottle-feeding:

1. Keep your baby's head in alignment with his body (maintain head, neck, and body in a straight line).

2. Do not allow your baby's head and neck to extend backward. Head and neck hyperextension can cause some irregular patterns to occur in your baby's mouth. These patterns include wide

jaw movements, excessive tongue protrusion, tongue humping or bunching, biting down for stability, and chomping.

3. Keep your baby's ear above his mouth, so fluid will not enter the Eustachian tubes. This means holding your baby upright at approximately a 45+ degree angle. As your child grows, he can be increasingly upright. This is crucial for bottle-fed babies. If your bottle-fed baby is positioned at 45 to 90 degrees to the horizon (Earth), then your bottle can be held even with the horizon (straight, not tipped up or down), so gravity does not make the liquid flow too fast. This process fits with paced (baby-led) bottle-feeding.

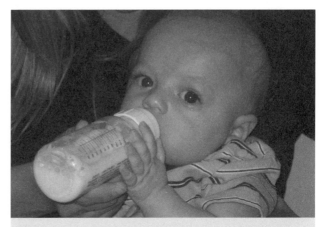

Photo 3.2: *Anthony (4 months) is sitting upright and making nice hand-mouth connections during paced (baby-led) bottle-feeding with his mom and Diane. His ears are above his mouth, so formula cannot enter his Eustachian tubes.*

4. Use paced (baby-led) bottle-feeding, which has some similarity to breastfeeding practices.[226] *The Breastfeeding Mother's Guide to Making More Milk* (2009), a book by Diana West and Lisa Marasco, contains detailed information on paced (baby-led) bottle-feeding.[227] You will also find videos online demonstrating this process. Your lactation consultant (preferably an IBCLC) can help you learn this technique.

   a. Stroke your baby's lips with the bottle nipple.

   b. Roll the bottle nipple into your baby's mouth when he opens the mouth demonstrating readiness to accept the nipple.

   c. Allow your baby a break between sucking bursts by tipping the bottle nipple slightly toward the mouth roof. Sucking bursts become longer as your baby ages.

   d. Use a slow-flow bottle nipple unless your lactation consultant (preferably an IBCLC) recommends a different flow to better match your own milk flow.

   e. Keep your baby's body upright at a 45- to 90-degree angle. The angle increases as your baby ages.

   f. Keep the bottle horizontal to reduce the effects of gravity on liquid flow, so your baby needs to suck the liquid from the bottle.

   g. Follow your baby's hunger cues to avoid overfeeding. These cues are discussed later in this chapter.

You might wonder, "Why is it a good idea to keep your baby's ear above his mouth when bottle-feeding?" While research is needed, it has long been suspected that babies who are bottle-fed lying down have a higher incidence of ear and sinus infections. This is related to the positioning of the Eustachian tubes, the sinuses, and gravity.

Eustachian tubes are positioned relatively horizontal in the newborn and become increasingly vertical as the child grows. Each Eustachian tube (one going to each ear) leads from the back of the nasopharynx (where the nasal area meets the throat) to the middle ear space behind the eardrum. Fluid is more likely to enter a baby's Eustachian tubes if the child is bottle-fed lying down, as gravity may pull the liquid downward into the middle ear. Eustachian tubes need to remain open to equalize pressure in the middle ear space.

If fluid from the bottle or stomach contents (due to reflux or spit up) enters the Eustachian tubes, it can travel into the middle ear space behind the eardrum. This space is essentially a sinus, as it is lined by mucous-producing membranes. If a foreign substance enters this area, more mucous is produced in the body's attempt to clear away the foreign substance. This mucous build-up in the middle ear space can become an ear infection.

When a full-term baby is born, a gelatinous substance[228] fills the middle ear space. However, this substance is absorbed during the first few weeks of life, leaving an open middle ear space. The middle ear contains three little bones that help the eardrum communicate sound to the inner ear. If the middle ear space is filled with fluid or infected mucous or the child's Eustachian tubes are closed, your child may have a significant hearing loss (such as a 30-decibel loss).[229][230] Conversational speech is approximately 65 decibels. Having a healthy middle ear is important for your child's hearing, speech, and language development.

Fluid in the middle ear, or Eustachian tube dysfunctions, can distort the way your child hears sounds. It may be most similar to when you hold your fingers in your ears or hear sounds while under water. When an airplane is descending, you can experience Eustachian tube closure and temporary hearing loss. Children are learning to discriminate the sounds of their own languages from birth.[231] Discriminating the different sounds of speech allows your child to learn speech and language. Therefore, your child's middle ears need to be kept clear from fluid and infection, and his Eustachian tubes need to remain open.

Sinus infections and rhinitis can also be caused by foreign matter such as reflux (commonly known as spit up) entering the nasal and sinus areas. Despite the cause, sinus infections or nasal congestion make it very difficult for your baby to breathe and feed. Most parents use a suctioning device to clear the baby's nose of excess mucous. As you know, good nasal breathing is essential for many health reasons, so it's important to keep your child's nose open for breathing. Speak with your child's pediatrician and/or pediatric ear, nose, and throat physician (otolaryngologist, ENT) for the best ways to clear your baby's nasal area and products (such as an appropriate nasal spray) to use.

When babies feed, they coordinate sucking, swallowing, and breathing in a sophisticated manner. A stuffy nose or closed Eustachian tubes may cause your baby to struggle with feeding, and he may compensate by taking an increasing number of breaths through his mouth. Long-term mouth breathing is unhealthy and makes it almost impossible to adequately coordinate sucking, swallowing, and breathing. By bottle-feeding your baby in an upright position (45- to 90-degree angle to the horizon, ear above mouth) with his head and body in alignment, you can help your child avoid ear, nasal, sinus, and other related problems.

What is Your Baby's Position During Breastfeeding or Bottle-Feeding?

Place check marks next to the description matching what your baby is doing and things you may want to change. Work with your lactation consultant (preferably an IBCLC) and/or other appropriate professional(s) on changes as needed.

WHAT YOU WANT MY BABY'S:	CHECK MARK	THINGS TO CHANGE MY BABY'S:	CHECK MARK
Head, neck, and body are aligned during feeding.	☐	Head and neck are turned or tipped too far back.	☐
Ear is at least slightly above the mouth during bottle-feeding (body and head upright at approximately a 45- to 90-degree angle to the Earth).	☐	Ear is not above the mouth because my baby is lying flat or at less than 45 to 90 degrees to the Earth during bottle-feeding.	☐
Body is in a correct laid-back, cradle or cross-cradle, side-lying position (belly-to-belly), or football position during breastfeeding.	☐	Head and neck are turned or tipped too far back.	☐
Nose is near the breast in most breast-feeding positions. Head and neck may be mildly extended (upward) with the chin into the breast and the nose free in the laid-back hold.	☐	Head and neck are tipped too far back.	☐
Baby has a wide, even, and sustained latch during breastfeeding and a graded, even latch during bottle-feeding.	☐	Baby has a poor latch on the breast or bottle.	☐

What Can Go Wrong in Breastfeeding or Bottle-Feeding?

A relatively flat roof of the mouth, adequate sucking or fat pads, tongue cupping, closeness or proximity of oral structures, as well as graded and coordinated jaw, lip, and tongue movement allow your young baby (birth to 4 months) to attain what therapists call *good intraoral pressure*.[232][233][234][235][236] Just like so many other systems in the body, the mouth is a pressure and valve system. Without the right pressure changes in the mouth, the liquid cannot move smoothly and easily to the throat for swallowing. This can cause your baby to work harder than necessary when feeding.

The roof of your young baby's mouth should be fairly flat, broad, and "U" shaped at birth, *not* high and *not* narrow. His sucking pads (balls of fat) should fill the cheek areas to hold the cheeks against the gums. His tongue should cup or groove around the bottle or breast nipple, *not* hump, bunch, or thrust. At the same time, the back of your baby's tongue moves appropriately to deliver the liquid easily from the breast or bottle to the throat for swallowing.

As you know, sucking or fat pads are balls of fat in a baby's cheeks that develop just before birth in a full-term baby (40 weeks gestation). They decrease in size between 4 and 6 months as your baby begins to chew and his cheeks become increasingly active along with his lips. Sucking pads provide side-stability while the mouth's roof (upper palate) and tongue provide upper and lower stability in the young infant's mouth during feeding.

Tongue humping or bunching (pushing up the middle of the tongue) means something has gone wrong in the mouth. Children who bunch their tongues to pump liquid from the bottle or breast are working too hard and fatigue easily. These babies may have inadequate sucking pads and/or cheek control. They may also have high, narrow palates and/or tongue ties. Babies seem to hump or bunch their tongues to attain the pressure changes needed in the mouth to move liquid toward the throat for swallowing. However, this compensation is not efficient or effective for feeding, as the liquid usually spills throughout the mouth instead of being carried in a stream through tongue cupping or grooving for swallowing.

Additionally, a baby's tongue should move over the lower gum during nutritive sucking and non-nutritive suckling. Babies whose tongues do not come out over the lower gum and lip to grasp and draw the breast into the mouth have difficulty breastfeeding. If a baby's tongue does not extend over the lower gum, he also tends to bite down or chomp on mom's nipples (ouch) or bottle nipples. Babies do this because the normal and natural bite reflex is triggered when the breast or bottle nipple come in contact with the front gums. Babies whose tongues do not move forward properly may have a tongue restriction, unstable jaw, and/or limited sucking pads.

However, some babies move their tongues too far forward (sometimes called a tongue thrust or exaggerated tongue protrusion). These babies usually work too hard to obtain milk from the breast or bottle. A tongue thrust is an *extensor pattern*, and it often goes along with heads and necks being extended too far back. Some babies may be doing this to open the airway. Think about cardio-pulmonary resuscitation (CPR), where the person's head and neck are extended back to open the airway. Another pattern often seen in babies who may be attempting to open the airway is a low and forward tongue position where the tongue is seen to rest between the lips. Low-resting tongue positions and tongue thrusting (exaggerated tongue protrusion) can become a lifelong pattern that is known to affect the development and shape of the airway, mouth, and teeth. High, narrow palates are often seen in conjunction with these problems.[237] Clinically, a low-resting tongue position and exaggerated tongue protrusion seem to be observed in more bottle-fed than breastfed babies. Babies with a low-resting tongue position and exaggerated tongue protrusion should be evaluated for potential tongue tie. See Tongue, Lip, and Buccal Restrictions section in Chapter 2.

Chomping, biting down, or excessive jaw movements during breastfeeding or bottle-feeding are not typical and may indicate the baby's mouth is unstable. In this situation, the infant seems to bite down in an attempt to stabilize the jaw, so he can move his lips and tongue. As you know, stability in the young infant's mouth during feeding is provided by the relatively flat upper palate, full set of sucking pads, close proximity of the oral structures, graded jaw movement (jaw moving just enough for the activity), adequate lip latch, and cupped tongue. Without this balance in the mouth, babies often develop compensatory patterns affecting the way they drink and swallow. These are maladaptive and require correction when possible. If such patterns are not corrected, children often require neuro-muscular re-education later in life known as *orofacial myofunctional treatment*.[238]

A baby should also have a good feeding rhythm. This means the entire mouth moves in a rhythmic manner. The nutritive suck (where your baby takes in breast milk or formula) occurs approximately 1 time per second. The non-nutritive suckle (a reflex) occurs about 2 times per second. As your baby becomes more skilled with the suck-swallow-breathe sequence, he will suck for longer periods of time without breaks. Breastfeeding or bottle-feeding should be a relatively quiet, smooth process. If your baby makes high-pitched, gulping, or other struggling sounds, the liquid may be flowing too quickly from the bottle or breast.

What is Your Baby Doing During Feeding?

Place check marks next to the description matching what your baby is doing and things you may want to change. Work with appropriate professionals such as a lactation consultant (preferably an IBCLC), feeding therapist (speech-language pathologist or occupational therapist who specializes in feeding), pediatrician, and/or others as needed.

WHAT YOU WANT MY BABY:	CHECK MARK	THINGS TO CHANGE MY BABY:	CHECK MARK
Has even, easy, and graded jaw movements when feeding (just enough movement for the activity).	☐	Has wide up-and-down jaw movements, biting, or chomping when feeding.	☐
Cups or grooves the tongue to conform to the shape of the bottle nipple or breast.	☐	Humps or bunches the tongue to get liquid from the bottle or breast.	☐

WHAT YOU WANT MY BABY: continued	CHECK MARK	THINGS TO CHANGE MY BABY: continued	CHECK MARK
Has even, graded, and appropriate tongue movement when feeding.	☐	Has tongue thrusting, exaggerated tongue protrusion, or a tongue restriction.	☐
Moves the tongue forward to grasp the breast (the tongue rides along with lower jaw when sucking) or has the tongue just over the lower gum when bottle-feeding.	☐	Cannot get the tongue over the lower gum, is thrusting the tongue out of the mouth, has a tongue restriction, and/or bites on the nipple.	☐
Has a good latch on the breast (wide and sustained) or bottle (jaw open just enough for the bottle nipple, lips evenly flared).	☐	Loses the latch frequently with air pockets or kissing sounds.	☐
Can draw liquid easily into the mouth.	☐	Works hard to draw in liquid.	☐
Has rhythmic and coordinated sucking, swallowing, and breathing during feeding.	☐	Makes gulping or struggling sounds, gasps for air, and/or does not have a good feeding rhythm.	☐

Choosing an Appropriate Bottle Nipple

Feeding is a nurturing and bonding process. Parents choose to bottle-feed exclusively or part-time for many reasons. Bottle-feeding allows Dad and others to take part in feeding the baby. It can give Mom a well-needed break and allow others to connect and bond with the baby. It also allows Mom to be away from the baby for an extended period of time without changing the baby's feeding schedule. As a feeding therapist, I prefer on-demand feeding when possible. If you bottle-feed your baby, review the information on paced (baby-led) bottle-feeding in a previous section of this chapter.

There are many steps in choosing the most appropriate bottle and nipple for your baby. The guidelines in this section of the book are meant to help you with the process. Choosing an appropriate bottle for your baby can be confusing because there are so many products on the market. This is likely because bottle-feeding is a medical way of feeding a baby. Companies are constantly trying to develop a bottle that works like the mom's breast or mimics the intraoral pressure the baby uses to pull the breast deeply into the mouth with good positioning and suction. No current baby bottle can do this.

Basically, you want a bottle nipple that fits your baby's mouth. If your baby has a small mouth, you will likely need a short, small nipple with an appropriate latch area. A child with a larger mouth may handle a longer nipple with a larger latch area. In my opinion, it's better to give your child a nipple that is a little too short than one that is too long. A nipple which is too long may encourage your baby to use incorrect movements, such as exaggerated tongue protrusion, that negatively affect mouth development. If your baby has difficulty maintaining a good latch on the bottle nipple, the nipple may be too long. If the bottle nipple is too long, it will often move in and out of your baby's mouth while she is drinking. This makes feeding inefficient and can tire your baby quickly. As previously mentioned, low-resting tongue position and tongue humping, bunching, or thrusting seem to be observed in more bottle-fed than breastfed babies. Babies with low-resting tongue position and irregular tongue movements should be evaluated for potential tongue tie. See Tongue, Lip, and Buccal Restrictions section in Chapter 2.

There is a simple test to determine if bottle nipple length is the problem or if your baby is having trouble getting enough pressure at the lips and inside the mouth to maintain the latch. Carefully support your baby's cheeks during bottle drinking. If the nipple stops moving in and out of your baby's mouth while the cheeks are properly supported, nipple length is not the problem. You will need to provide your baby with appropriately and carefully applied cheek support until she learns to use the muscles of her jaw, cheeks, and lips to maintain the latch. This is what therapists call a *motor plan*. Your baby may learn this quickly, so you may not need to support her cheeks for long (just until she learns to keep the cheeks near the side gums when feeding).

Appropriately applied cheek support means you only give your baby the support needed to effectively and efficiently feed. This is a dance. Cheeks activate lips. So, you will place your thumb near the center of one cheek, and your index or middle finger near the center of her other cheek. The angle of your hand is under her chin. You press gently inward on the cheek tissue and pull your fingers forward slightly to help activate your baby's lips. Be careful not to squeeze your baby's cheeks too tightly or glide your fingers over the cheek tissue. This can cause liquid to flow very quickly into and though your baby's mouth, overwhelming her airway. If this happens, you will hear coughing, high-pitched gulping sounds, or other abnormal sounds during feeding. Once your baby learns the motor plan for bringing her cheeks toward the gums, you will no longer need to provide cheek support.

Prudently applied cheek support helps babies born with thin or missing sucking pads and those with poor muscle tone in their cheeks attain the oral pressure needed to feed effectively. You may also see your baby's tongue cup (along with the cheek support) because you are now providing the lateral stability your child needs to suck properly. However, if the bottle nipple continues to move in and out of your baby's mouth when you provide careful cheek support, you need to find a nipple that fits your baby's mouth. Product labeling can be misleading. Your child may require a nipple that is labeled differently than you would expect. For example, some nipples are labeled *preemie*, *newborn*, or *mini*, but may be a perfect nipple size for your baby. This does not say anything about your baby's development, except she may require a certain nipple that appropriately fits her mouth. Like the saying goes, "There is a key for every lock." Finding the right key is important.

Nipple shape can be another consideration when choosing a bottle nipple for your baby. Many nipples are rounded so the tongue can cup around them. I prefer these because they encourage tongue cupping. This is particularly important for the newborn baby who uses a deeply-cupped tongue while drinking. However, some babies drink better from what may be identified as an orthodontic nipple. These nipples may encourage up-down front of tongue movement, but no bottle nipple is likely orthodontic in nature. As previously discussed, bottle-feeding is a different process than breastfeeding. Breastfeeding is the best way to keep a baby's mouth in shape from birth.[239]

A good latch means your baby's lips maintain a hold on the latch area of the bottle nipple. The latch area is the part of the bottle nipple that flares out from the nipple itself. A wide latch area may encourage better mouth development. However, much research is needed in the area of bottle-feeding and mouth development. Most current research discusses the detriments of bottle-feeding and the value of breastfeeding for mouth development.

If your baby is using an appropriately sized bottle nipple and still has difficulty maintaining a latch, your baby may have a jaw weakness or some other difficulty you may not be able to determine on your own. Consult with a feeding specialist if you need help with this process (IBCLC and/or feeding therapist). As previously mentioned, providing your baby with carefully applied cheek support can help your baby appropriately compensate for a weak latch until the difficulty is resolved. There are specific activities to address jaw weakness in the book *Nobody Ever Told Me (or My Mother) That! Everything from Bottles and Breathing to Healthy Speech Development* by Diane Bahr.

If you have ongoing questions or concerns about the right bottle nipple for your baby or your baby's latch on the nipple, work with a professional. Appropriately trained occupational therapists, speech-language pathologists, lactation consultants, nurse practitioners, and some pediatricians can help you with this process. Check with the hospital where you delivered your baby or hospitals that specialize in feeding to find professionals who can help you. Here are a few resources for finding feeding professionals and feeding information:

RESOURCES	WEBSITES
Feeding Matters	www.feedingmatters.org
New Visions	www.new-vis.com
The International Lactation Consultant Association	www.ilca.org
The United States Lactation Consultant Association	uslca.org
The American Speech-Language-Hearing Association	www.asha.org
The American Occupational Therapy Association	www.aota.org

Choosing the Right Bottle Nipple for Your Baby

Place check marks next to the description matching any problems you are having and things you may want to try. Work with appropriate professionals such as a lactation consultant (preferably an IBCLC), feeding therapist (speech-language pathologist or occupational therapist who specializes in feeding), pediatrician, and/or others as needed.

PROBLEM	CHECK MARK	THINGS TO TRY	CHECK MARK
My baby's tongue does not cup around the bottle nipple.	☐	Choose a rounded nipple rather than the orthodontic-type nipple.	☐
The bottle nipple moves in and out of my baby's mouth.	☐	Carefully provide cheek support.	☐
The bottle nipple moves in and out of my baby's mouth when I give appropriate cheek support.	☐	Try a shorter nipple, even if the packaging is labeled for a younger baby.	☐

What to Do if Your Baby has Difficulty Maintaining a Latch

Maintaining a good latch on the bottle or breast is a common problem. As mentioned previously, it's important to check nipple size and shape if you are bottle-feeding. Also, pay attention to your baby's positioning. If your baby's head and body are out of alignment, this can significantly affect the latch. Your baby's head, shoulders, and hips should be in fairly straight line.

If you are breastfeeding, and your baby is having difficulty maintaining a latch, see your lactation consultant (preferably an IBCLC) for an assessment as soon as possible. The lactation consultant will evaluate your baby's mouth for many of the problems we discuss in this book and can recommend needed specialists. In my practice, I rely on lactation consultants to send me appropriate referrals and to help the family follow through with my recommendations. We work hand-in-hand with other professionals as needed in a team approach.

When working with your baby's latch, you may need to provide her with some carefully applied cheek support whether breastfeeding or bottle-feeding. This can be a temporary measure to assist your baby in maintaining the lateral (or side) stability needed in her mouth and bringing her lips forward to suck correctly. Proper cheek support can help your baby create an appropriate amount of intraoral mouth pressure to draw in liquid from the bottle or breast easily and efficiently.

To provide appropriate cheek support, place your thumb on one of your baby's cheeks and index or middle finger on the other. Press gently but firmly inward toward your baby's gums while pulling your fingers slightly forward toward your baby's lips. Do not slide your fingers over your baby's skin in any direction. You will see your baby's lips flare because the muscles of the cheeks help to move the lips. You may also see your baby's tongue cup because you are now providing the lateral stability your child needs to suck properly.

For many years, lactation consultants have taught moms the dancer hand position. This is where the mom supports the baby's cheeks and chin with her free hand while the baby is breastfeeding. Many moms have found this hold difficult to maintain, particularly when using a cross-cradle (cross-over) breastfeeding position. Therefore, a breastfeeding position change may be needed. It can be easier to use the dancer hold in a cradle, side-lying, or laid-back breastfeeding position.

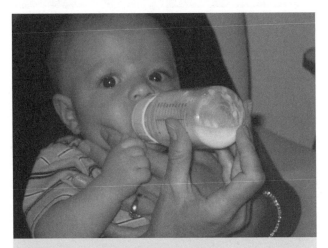

Photo 3.3: *Anthony (4 months) demonstrates carefully applied cheek support with Diane. Properly applied cheek support is often needed for breastfeeding babies when they are born without a complete set of sucking or fat pads in their cheeks (such as preemies or close-to-term babies). In breastfed babies, this is called the dancer hand position. However, some bottle-fed children may also need correctly applied cheek support if they don't have enough intra oral pressure to feed properly from a bottle.*

Modified cheek support can be used with the cross-cradle hold. Gravity is often the culprit in this situation, as gravity pulls the lower cheek toward the center of the Earth. Therefore, the lower cheek does not remain against your baby's gum surface during breastfeeding. Appropriate pressure in the mouth is lost when this occurs. Breastfeeding moms using a cross-cradle hold can apply gentle but firm pressure to the baby's lower cheek surface to help the baby compensate for this difficulty.

You can also give your baby a little jaw support along with cheek support when needed. Place the area of your hand between your thumb and index finger under your baby's chin to support the jaw. However, it's essential you do not stop your baby's jaw from moving up-and-down or force her jaw to move in an unnatural direction. Providing jaw and cheek support is like dancing smoothly with a partner.

Properly applied cheek and jaw support can help your baby to latch. However, these are usually temporary measures. Your baby may have a subtle difficulty in the mouth causing the latching concern. Subtle concerns are often problematic because they can be difficult to identify. This is a good reason to seek help from a feeding specialist such as a lactation consultant (preferably an IBCLC) and/or feeding therapist (typically a speech-language pathologist or occupational therapist who specializes in feeding).

Helping Your Baby Latch Onto the Breast or Bottle

Place check marks next to the description matching any problems you are having and things you may want to try. Work with appropriate professionals such as a lactation consultant (preferably an IBCLC), feeding therapist (speech-language pathologist or occupational therapist who specializes in feeding), pediatrician, and/or others as needed.

PROBLEM	CHECK MARK	THINGS TO TRY	CHECK MARK
Your baby is not latching properly on the bottle (lips not latched to the flared part of nipple).	☐	Provide carefully applied cheek support using thumb and index or middle finger; check nipple length if this does not work.	☐
Your baby is not latching properly on the breast (breast should be drawn deeply into your baby's mouth with a wide and sustained lip latch).	☐	— When using cross-cradle, cradle, or side-lying positions, carefully provided cheek support may be given to the lower cheek (modified dancer hand position). — When using cradle, laid-back, or side-lying positions, cheek support using thumb and index or middle finger may be given (dancer hand position). You will need to switch hands as you switch sides for feeding so a hand is free to provide support. Jaw support may be provided if needed.	☐

What to Do if Liquid is Flowing Too Fast or Too Slowly

The best way to tell if liquid is flowing too fast from the breast or bottle is to listen for the sounds your baby makes while feeding. Mom's breast milk can let down very quickly, or fluid can flow through the bottle nipple too fast. When this occurs, your baby may make little high-pitched, gulping sounds. Your baby's vocal cords are making the high-pitched sound while closing to keep liquid from going into the airway. You may also hear little struggling sounds like your baby is trying to clear her throat. This means your baby is working too hard and may be penetrating or aspirating fluid into her airway. If your baby is gasping for breath, there is definitely a problem.

If you hear any of these sounds, find a way to slow the flow. For quick let down while breastfeeding, place your baby into a more upright position to limit the effects of gravity. The laid-back breastfeeding position works very well for this problem. Side-lying can be a helpful position as it also limits the effects of gravity. Your lactation consultant (preferably an IBCLC) can help you with this process.

For bottle-fed babies, flow can be controlled to match your baby's suck by choosing the correct bottle nipple. Some nipples flow more slowly than others. Slow-flow nipples are usually recommended for paced (baby-led) bottle-feeding. This method is particularly suggested for babies who are concurrently breastfeeding and bottle-feeding. Although, your lactation consultant (preferably an IBCLC) may suggest a bottle nipple flow that best matches your breast milk flow. Paced (baby-led) bottle-feeding is a good method for most bottle-fed babies.

There are variable-flow nipples where the flow can be adjusted according to your baby's sucking ability. Variable-flow nipples allow liquid to flow more slowly if your baby is gasping, gulping, or struggling in any way. They also permit liquid to flow faster as your baby develops more skill. If your baby has a weak suck, the variable-flow nipple will allow your baby an easier flow until her suck is stronger. You can actually assist your baby in developing a stronger suck by having her work a little harder (but not to the point of fatigue) as you change the flow of the nipple over time. Work with a lactation consultant (preferably an IBCLC) or feeding therapist (speech-language pathologist or occupational therapist who specializes in feeding) on this process.

Important Note for Parents Who Are Bottle-Feeding

Please do not modify the bottle nipple your baby uses from its original design. Some parents have enlarged bottle nipple holes for a faster flow. Nipples that flow too fast can cause significant mouth development and swallowing problems. Some parents have cut the nipple so formula mixed with cereal can come through the bottle nipple. Cereal is best presented from a spoon or open cup when the time is right, and your baby can appropriately manage it from the spoon or open cup. If your baby has trouble drinking from a nipple, try different nipples. However, this process can be a bit overwhelming because there are so many bottles on the market. Therefore, you may need a feeding professional to help you.

I like the story of *The Three Bears* when we talk about liquid flow. We want liquid flow from the breast or bottle to be *just right* for your baby. If liquid flows too fast, it can cause your baby to cough or choke. Some babies learn to pull their tongues back to protect the airway from the fast-flowing liquid. This is a hard habit to break. If liquid flows too slowly, your baby may hump and/or thrust the tongue to apply more pressure. The greatest concern about inappropriate liquid flow is your baby can develop incorrect feeding habits that can affect her swallowing for a lifetime.

Liquid Flow from the Breast or Bottle

Place check marks next to the description matching any problems you are having and things you may want to try or do. Work with appropriate professionals such as a lactation consultant (preferably an

IBCLC), feeding therapist (speech-language pathologist or occupational therapist who specializes in feeding), pediatrician, and/or others as needed.

PROBLEM	CHECK MARK	THINGS TO TRY/DO	CHECK MARK
Breastfeeding: Milk let down too fast.	☐	Feed your baby more upright (laid-back position) or in side-lying; work with your lactation consultant (preferably an IBCLC).	☐
Bottle nipple flows too fast.	☐	Change nipple to a slow-flow nipple and use paced (baby-led) bottle-feeding. Consider a variable-flow nipple if needed. Work with your lactation consultant and/or feeding therapist.	☐
Bottle nipple flows too slow.	☐	Change nipple to a faster-flow nipple and use paced (baby-led) bottle feeding. Consider a variable-flow nipple if needed. Work with your lactation consultant and/or feeding therapist.	☐
Difficulty finding correct nipple flow.	☐	Consult a feeding professional for help.	☐

Nutrition and Hydration

There are many good resources on nutrition. This book is not meant to replace them but to lead you in the direction of appropriate information. Here are some resources on nutrition in addition to the information your child's pediatrician and registered pediatric dietician or nutritionist may provide:

RESOURCES	WEBSITES
Academy of Nutrition and Dietetics	www.eatright.org
American Academy of Pediatrics	www.aap.org and www.healthychildren.org
Ellyn Satter Institute	www.ellynsatterinstitute.org
Nutrition.gov	www.nutrition.gov

Good nutrition is difficult to attain if your baby's mouth and digestive system are not working well. You now know a lot about how your baby's mouth works. Let's talk about some basics of nutrition.

Appropriate weight gain is essential. This means your baby should not be overweight or underweight. Breastfed infants are seldom overweight because they stop eating when they are full. "Sometimes they eat bigger meals, and sometimes they snack."[240] The mom's breast milk production adjusts to her baby's nutritional needs when breastfeeding is going well. Therefore, the mom's nutrition and hydration are important for the baby's nutrition and hydration. Work with your lactation consultant (preferably an IBCLC) on providing you and your baby with the best possible breastfeeding experience. Here are some resources to help you.

RESOURCES	WEBSITES
American Academy of Pediatrics	www.aap.org and www.healthychildren.org
Breast and Bottle-Feeding	www.breastandbottlefeeding.com
Breastfeeding Help Desk	www.breastfeedinghelpdesk.com
Kellymom, Parenting and Breastfeeding	kellymom.com
La Leche League	www.lalecheleague.org
Nurturing Naturally	www.nurturingnaturallylc.net
World Health Organization	www.who.int/en

It's a little trickier to judge whether a bottle-fed baby is getting appropriate nutrition. This is likely one reason some bottle-fed babies may be overfed. As a therapist, I have worked with many babies who continued drinking from and sucking on a bottle for apparent comfort after their nutritional needs were apparently met.

Bottle-fed babies also tend to have more problems with excessive spit up, technically called *gastroesophageal reflux*. Breastfed babies do not seem to have this problem as often because the mom's milk supply adjusts to her baby's nutritional needs. In general, babies also digest breast milk better than formula.

A baby's stomach is very small (about the size of her fist). If a baby overfills her stomach even by a half an ounce, this can contribute to gastroesophageal reflux (spit up) and discomfort. You know how it feels to over eat. If you suffer from reflux, you also recognize you are more likely to experience reflux if you overfill your stomach. Both breast-fed and bottle-fed babies need to self-regulate the amount they eat according to their own needs. It's crucial to allow your baby to decide how much and how often to eat unless she is demonstrating signs of poor growth and/or de-hydration.

Your baby will also go through some growth spurts, so some days she will be hungrier than others. According to Ellyn Satter, some pre-dictable growth spurts occur at 7 to 10 days, 5 to 6 weeks, and 3 months of age.[241] Feeding amounts will vary during these times. If you become concerned about your baby's growth or weight gain, work with your child's pedia-trician, lactation consultant (preferably an IB-

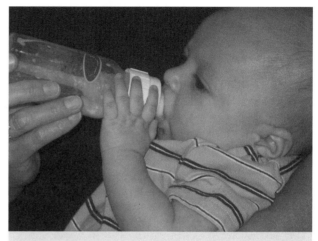

Photo 3.4: *Anthony (4 months) has a nice even lip latch on the bottle even when getting sleepy. His hand is on the bottle for the hand-mouth connection. Anthony's body language communicates he is sleepy and likely finished eating.*

CLC), and registered pediatric dietician or nutritionist when needed. The best way to track your baby's growth is through frequent weight and measurement checks. Pediatricians' offices and most lactation consultants have scales and measurement equipment available. You can rent or buy an infant scale if it's more convenient to have one at home.

Your child's pediatrician, lactation consultant (preferably an IBCLC), and/or registered pediatric di-etician or nutritionist will have growth charts to help you track increases in your baby's weight, head circumference, and length. Many nutrition resources contain these charts as well. Ask your child's pediatrician to use growth charts developed by the World Health Organization if you are breastfeed-ing because some other growth charts are based on formula-fed babies. Formula-fed babies grow somewhat differently than breastfed babies. There are also apps with growth charts developed by the World Health Organization and the Centers for Disease Control and Prevention.

As you know, many parents are anxious about their child's nutrition. This can cause some parents to err on the side of overfeeding. While I think this concern is perfectly normal, it often causes prob-lems with weight and feeding later on. If you are nervous about how much your baby is eating, your baby can sense your feelings. This makes feeding stressful for you and for your baby. I want you to be relaxed and confident when you feed your baby. Get good information on nutrition and how your child is growing.

Children tend to eat what they need and self-limit the amount of food they take. Parents need to learn their baby's body language and communication signals to know when their baby is full.

What My Baby's Body is Telling Me

In this chart, you find Ellyn Satter's information on baby body language.[242] Place check marks in the column next to the description matching what your baby is doing.

READY TO EAT	CHECK MARK
Eyes open wider than usual.	☐
Face looks bright.	☐
Arms and legs curled over belly.	☐
Touch around mouth results in a rooting reflex and/or mouthing.	☐
Baby may suck on hands.	☐
Fussing is a last resort.	☐
READY TO TAKE A BREAK	
May pause to rest.	☐
May pause to look at you and/or socialize.	☐
HOW TO TELL WHEN YOUR BABY IS FULL, OR SOMETHING DOES NOT FEEL RIGHT	
Sucking slows down.	☐
Baby lets go of the nipple.	☐
Baby will turn away.	☐
Baby will begin to kick, squirm, arch back, or get fussy if you don't pay attention to the signals listed above.	☐

Remember, the amount your baby eats is individual and is based on her own metabolism and stomach size. Age, growth rate, and activity level also factor into this equation.[243] Breast milk and formula usually contain adequate water, so you *won't give your baby extra water* until around 6 months of age (unless otherwise directed by your baby's pediatrician). The pediatrician and lactation consultant (preferably an IBCLC) will guide you in the amounts of fluid (breast milk or formula) your baby needs as she grows.

There are iron-fortified formulas for babies. Have your child's pediatrician check to see if your baby needs extra iron. Also, if you are using a powdered formula you mix with water, have your water tested for lead and other contaminants. It is best to boil the water you mix with formula for 3 minutes during your baby's first 6 months of life.[244] Check with your child's pediatrician on the safety of using powdered formula, as there have been recalls on powdered formula. Pre-made liquid formula is said to have less risk of contamination than powdered formulas.

The water your baby gets through breast milk or formula does a lot for your baby's body. Seventy-five percent of the body and 85 percent of the brain is water.[245][246] Water "regulates all functions of the body."[247] It helps to keep body chemistry in balance by carrying hormones, nutrients, and other important substances to the cells of the body. Water also removes waste from these cells. *Do not* give your baby extra water before 6 months unless directed by your child's pediatrician.

Adequate hydration is connected to immune system function. Dehydration leads to disease. Some signs or symptoms of dehydration can include chronic drowsiness, chronic pain, constipation, belly pain, head pain, stress, depression, chronic upper respiratory illness, asthma, allergies, excessive body weight, diabetes, and problems with sleep.[248]

The following may lead to or indicate poor growth and dehydration in your baby:[249]

- Decrease in "pees and poops"
- Few feedings
- Decrease in number of feedings
- Overly sleepy
- Weak suck
- Little interest in feeding

Here are some signs of significant dehydration. Please contact your baby's physician immediately and take your baby to the emergency room if you see these signs.[250]

- Dry mouth and decreased "pees"
- Sunken eyes with few tears when crying

- Sunken soft spot

- Tight, dry skin

- Fast pulse and breathing

- Skin unusually blue

- Cold hands and/or feet

- Listlessness, drowsiness, or unconsciousness

4

Good Spoon-Feeding, Cup-Drinking, Straw-Drinking, and Chewing Practices, and What to Do If Problems Arise

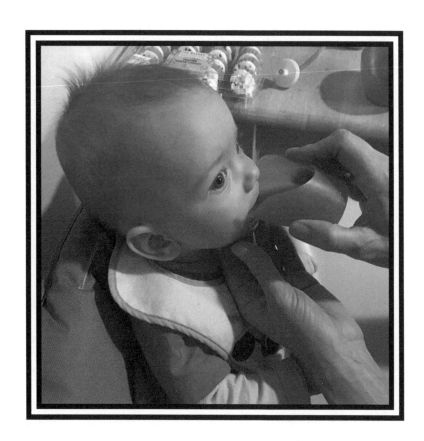

When your baby is 6 months of age, you will begin to introduce new foods and liquids. You do not want to overwhelm yourself or your baby, so you have to make some choices. Ask yourself, "What do I feel most comfortable introducing to my baby first? Spoon-feeding, drinking from an open cup, drinking from a straw, or taking bites and chewing?" Your baby is ready for all of these processes around 6 months. Therefore, you can introduce them within weeks of one another. Remember, it only takes 2 to 3 weeks of daily practice to develop a new habit. And, feeding, eating, and drinking is something we do several times each day.

Your choice many depend on the culture in which you live. Many parents in Westernized societies choose to begin by teaching their babies spoon-feeding or open cup-drinking around 6 months of age because it is customary. After that, they may choose to teach straw-drinking or taking bites of food for chewing. This way, all of these skills can be taught within a relatively short period of time. If you live in a different culture, you may choose a different process for feeding your baby as determined by your culture.

Appropriate spoon-feeding, cup- and straw-drinking, taking bites of food, and *particularly chewing* at the back molar areas encourages the best mouth development possible. These feeding skills can be taught *in any order you choose* around 6 months. If you are using baby-led weaning, you may want to begin with a soft baby cookie or other appropriate, soft food held by you and your child (speak with your child's pediatrician about what to introduce). If you are breastfeeding, you may decide to begin with open cup-drinking, since this process seems most similar to breastfeeding. Ultimately, *taking safe bites and chewing* is essential for the best possible jaw development. Good mouth development supports adequate nutrition through effective food and liquid management and good digestion.

Digestion begins in the mouth. Saliva contains enzymes that begin to break down food, so it can be metabolized by the body. Chewing food for a sufficient amount of time mixes it with saliva. We should chew each bite of food 20 or more times when possible. Your child will develop this ability as he learns to take bites of and chew foods of increasing texture. See Chapter 1 for Food and Liquid Introduction Checklist: Birth to 24 Months.

The methods discussed in this book, in conjunction with the ones you have learned in your baby's first 5 or 6 months of life, can also reduce the need for orthodontics (such as a palatal expander or braces) later on. If your child does require orthodontics at some point, you can minimize the work needed by helping your child develop the best mouth structures possible through good feeding and mouthing experiences. See Appropriate Mouth Items and Toys in a later section of this chapter.

It may take a little time and practice for you and your baby to learn the feeding skills discussed in this book. However, the techniques are easy to apply and can make feeding fun. In the long run, they save you time and aggravation. You are going to feed your baby anyway, so why not make it a pleasurable and successful experience? Dr. Harvey Karp says parents who succeed in feeding and calming their babies "feel proud, confident, and on top of the world!"[251]

As you and your baby learn the exciting new skills taught in this book, think about how you learn any new skill (such as a tennis serve, a golf swing, key-boarding, or ballroom dancing). You need a certain amount of consistent practice and repetition to develop these abilities. This is the same process you will use when you and your baby are learning the feeding dance. As feeding partners, you will both be learning new skills to help you feel happy, satisfied, and successful.

Positioning Your Baby for New Feeding Activities

If you begin spoon-feeding or open cup-drinking with your baby before 6 months of age, your baby will usually not be sitting up on her own. As discussed previously, you will only begin feeding your baby prior to 6 months of age *if recommended by your child's pediatrician*. You can begin spoon-feeding or open cup-drinking with your baby placed securely in a baby seat if your baby is not yet sitting up. The baby seat can be placed on a secure table or countertop, and you can sit at eye level with your baby. However, *do not leave your baby unsupervised* in this position. It's important to position your baby so you are sitting eye-to-eye. This allows you to make appropriate eye contact, keep your baby's head and neck in a good position, and communicate with your baby.

If your head is above your baby's head during feeding, your baby will look up at you to make eye contact. This can place your baby's head and neck into excessive extension (too far back). Remember when you learned Cardio Pulmonary Resuscitation (CPR), how you extended the person's head and neck to open the airway? We don't want your baby's airway open too wide during feeding because this may cause coughing or choking.

If you feed your baby by standing or sitting above her (called *bird feeding*), you are requiring her to open her airway. This makes swallowing more difficult to control and places your baby at risk for aspiration or choking. It also encourages extension patterns in the mouth, such as wide jaw movements and exaggerated tongue protrusion (sometimes called tongue thrusting). These movements can cause your child problems later in life. As previously mentioned, low-resting tongue position and exaggerated tongue protrusion seem to be observed more often in bottle-fed than breastfed babies.

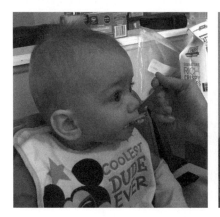 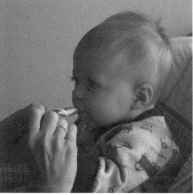

Photo 4.1: *Cannon (6.5 months) and Anthony (12 months) are sitting at eye level with Diane while eating from a small Maroon Spoon. This places both boy's heads into a neutral position for spoon-feeding. Anthony is helping Diane bring the spoon to his mouth.*

Babies with low-resting tongue positions and exaggerated tongue protrusions should be evaluated for potential tongue tie. See Tongue, Lip, and Buccal Restrictions section in Chapter 2.

By 6 months of age, most babies will be sitting on their own. However, many of the high chairs on the market are a too large for many babies. I prefer the Keekaroo, the STOKKE Tripp Trapp chair, the Svan Signet, or other similar chairs because they provide excellent postural support, can be adjusted as your child grows, and you can feed your baby at eye level.

How Is Your Baby Positioned During Feeding?

Place check marks in the columns next to the description matching what your baby is doing and things you may want to change.

WHAT YOU WANT MY BABY IS:	CHECK MARK	THINGS TO CHANGE MY BABY IS:	CHECK MARK
Sitting in an appropriate baby seat with her body upright at a 45- to 90-degree angle to the Earth (before 6 months of age or sitting up).	☐	Not sitting in a stable seat with her body upright at a 45- to 90-degree angle to the Earth (before 6 months of age or sitting up).	☐
Sitting in a chair that fits my baby and is properly adjusted.	☐	Not sitting well supported in a chair with her body upright at a 90-degree angle to the Earth.	☐
Looking straight into my eyes when we are feeding.	☐	Looking up at me when we are feeding.	☐

Jaw Support

In addition to placing your child into a supported position for feeding, you might find jaw support helpful during initial spoon-feeding, open cup-drinking, or straw-drinking. Provide jaw stability with your non-dominant hand (left-hand if you are right-handed or right-hand if you are left-handed). Never force or push on your baby's jaw in any direction, as this can hurt your baby. Instead, hold her jaw like you would hold a dance partner, and allow your baby's jaw to move naturally. Your baby is taking the lead in this dance, and you are following. Jaw support can help both of you feel more secure when learning new feeding skills.

As you face your baby at eye-to-eye level, you can stabilize your baby's jaw with your non-dominant hand in a couple of ways. One way is to place your index finger under the bony part of your baby's chin and your thumb on her chin. Another way is to place your thumb and index finger along your baby's jawbone. Then use your dominant hand (right if you are right-handed or left if you are left-handed) to feed your baby using the methods discussed in the next sections of the book. Jaw

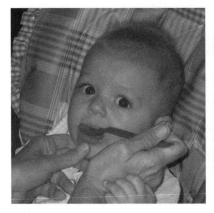
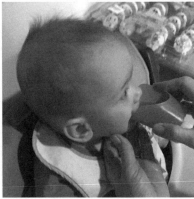

Photo 4.2: *Anthony (6 months) receives some jaw support while learning to eat from a small Maroon Spoon. Cannon (6.5 months) receives some jaw support while learning to drink from a small pink cut-out cup.*

support can help both you and your baby feel more comfortable and organized while learning these new feeding skills. Your baby will also feel less vulnerable because you are providing some calming touch before moving toward her mouth with a spoon, open cup, or straw.

Spoon-Feeding

Before you feed your baby with a spoon, see how you use a spoon in your own mouth. Get some applesauce, yogurt, pudding, or another soft food you like to eat. Observe how you take the food off of the spoon and what you do with the food after you take it from the spoon. This exercise will give you more awareness regarding how the mouth works.

How Do You Eat From a Spoon?

Place an answer next to the question. Take a spoonful of applesauce or another soft food and notice the following.

QUESTIONS	YOUR ANSWERS
Do you open your jaw really wide or just enough for the spoon?	
Do your lips help to take the food from the spoon?	

QUESTIONS	YOUR ANSWERS
Is your tongue completely under the spoon, or is your tongue tip grasping and guiding the spoon?	
How far do you place the spoon into your mouth?	
Do you place the spoon straight into your mouth or at an angle?	

If you tipped the spoon handle upward when you removed it from your mouth, you probably had a spoon with a bowl that was too deep. This is a very common problem with adult spoons that, fortunately, some baby spoons do not have. Most people place the spoon partially (½ to ¾ of the spoon depending on the size of the spoon) into the mouth. Your tongue may come forward to grasp and guide the spoon into your mouth. Once you remove the food from the spoon with your lips, you manage the food within your mouth, and then your tongue gathers the food centrally to move it back for the swallow.

The spoon is often inserted at an angle (up to 45 degrees from the left or right) depending on which hand you normally use to feed yourself. Most people place a reasonable amount of food on the spoon, so the lips can work to remove the food from the spoon. The jaw, lips, and cheeks provide the primary actions in removing food from the spoon (with the jaw opening just enough for the spoon and the lips and cheeks working together to take food from the spoon).

How to Properly Spoon-Feed Your Baby

Up to this point, your baby has hopefully used a coordinated suck, swallow, and breathe pattern to manage formula or breast milk. Taking food from a spoon is very different than taking liquid from the bottle or breast.

Many parents begin spoon-feeding with baby cereal. For successful early spoon-feeding you can:

- Begin by mixing baby cereal with water, formula, or breast milk, so it is not too thick, sticky, or runny—just right.

- Help your baby become accustomed to the taste and texture of the cereal by dipping your clean or gloved finger into the cereal and giving her tastes from your finger. Or, let your baby dip her finger(s) into the food and place them into her mouth.

- Help your baby become accustomed to the spoon by letting her hold and mouth the spoon with your assistance. Hands and mouths are meant to work together. There are baby dipper spoons she can hold and dip into foods, such as the Num Num or ChooMee dipper spoons.

- Begin spoon-feeding by dipping the spoon into the cereal mixture and letting your baby taste the cereal from the tip of the spoon, rather than placing a typical amount of food on the spoon at first.

- When you place more food on the spoon, your baby's tongue protrusion reflex (likely part of the suckling reflex) may push some of the food out. Don't worry about this. It will take you and your baby a little time to learn the new habit of spoon-feeding. Eventually, the front of your baby's tongue may grasp the spoon like the breast and guide the spoon into the mouth.

Here are some characteristics of good spoon-feeding:

- Use a small, flat-bowled spoon that fits your baby's lip area comfortably (the *small* Maroon Spoon works well for this).

- Place a small and/or reasonable amount of food on the spoon.

- Place the spoon into her mouth only far enough, so the food will be removed as her jaw and lips close.

- Do not use your baby's upper lip or gum to scrape food off of the spoon. If you find yourself doing this, slow down. Food should be removed by jaw and lip closure, so there is no need for the spoon to be tipped upward.

Be sure the spoon fits your baby's mouth. Regular, adult-sized spoons are too large. The bowls of those spoons are too deep for your baby's mouth. There are many small spoons with relatively flat bowls available.

My favorite spoon is the *small* Maroon Spoon. It has a small flat bowl, allowing the baby to close the jaw and remove the food with his or her lips. It is also widely used all over the world with children who have special feeding concerns. However, don't let this deter you from using the *small* Maroon Spoon. It's a wonderful, easy-to-use spoon. See the following list for information on where to purchase *small* Maroon Spoons and other feeding tools.

Companies that carry feeding products for children that cannot be found in most stores:

COMPANIES	WEBSITES
ARK Therapeutic Services, Inc.	www.arktherapeutic.com
SuperDuper Publications	www.superduperinc.com
TalkTools	www.talktools.com
Therapro	www.theraproducts.com

At 6 months of age, your baby can close her lips on the spoon if you allow sufficient time. Over the next few months, she will begin to move her lips, cheeks, and tongue independently of her jaw. Independent lip, cheek, tongue, and jaw movement is essential for the development of increasingly sophisticated eating, drinking, and speaking skills. Babies who do not learn these skills often have difficulty removing food from the spoon, leaving a lot of extra food on the lips. However, if your baby has a little bit of food on her lips, don't scrape or wipe it off unless needed. By having some food left on her lips, she will learn to move her lips and tongue to remove the food as she develops. The lip sound "m" is frequently heard when babies begin spoon-feeding. This may be one reason we say "mmm" when something tastes good.

Your baby's lips and cheeks will become progressively active over time, with development and the use of good feeding techniques. By 6 months of age, your baby's sucking or fat pads should have disappeared from her cheeks. Around 3 to 4 months of age, babies begin chewing on hands, fingers, and appropriate mouth toys (see section on Appropriate Mouth Items and Toys found later in this chapter). Therefore, chewing begins to replace sucking and cheek pads are no longer needed. Increasingly

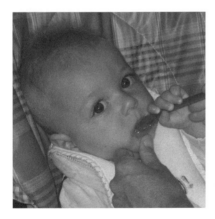
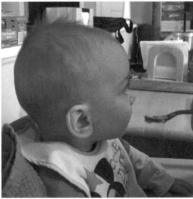

Photo 4.3: *Anthony (6 months) helps to bring the small Maroon Spoon to his mouth. Cannon (6.5 months) just cleared the small Maroon Spoon with his lips.*

mature lip movements will become apparent around 8 months of age as your baby uses her upper lip to remove the food from the spoon.

When you spoon-feed your baby, place a small and/or reasonable amount of food on the spoon. Be careful not to overload it. A reasonable amount of food allows your baby to discriminate or feel the amount of food on the spoon and manage the food appropriately. Your baby can experience the texture, size, and shape of food. This oral discrimination is needed for the effective manipulation of food and liquid within the mouth. Discriminative mouthing begins around 5 to 6 months of age. This discrimination is used in eating, drinking, and speaking.

If you place too much food into your baby's mouth at one time, your baby may have difficulty learning to manage spoon foods well. During spoon-feeding, we want your baby to practice graded (just enough) jaw, lip, and cheek use, as well as good tongue movement for swallowing. These are precursors of a mature swallowing pattern which emerges around 11 to 12 months of age. Now, let's learn a couple effective spoon-feeding methods.

We will first learn natural spoon-feeding. This is how you feed yourself.

1. Place the front portion of the spoon straight into your baby's mouth. Allow the bottom of the spoon to touch your baby's lower lip. Do not place the spoon too far into your baby's mouth. Remember how far you typically place the spoon into your mouth.

2. When the spoon is placed on your baby's lower lip, wait for your baby's top lip to come down and close on the spoon. Once your baby's upper lip closes on the spoon, remove the spoon from your baby's mouth in a level manner. You will be pulling the spoon horizontally (straight out) from your baby's mouth.

Important Note: Do not tip the spoon upward to scrape the food off of your baby's upper lip or gum. Babies who are fed in this way are not learning to use their lips to effectively manipulate food and often have difficulty learning to use their lips properly at a later age. You can see some adults whose upper lips do not close or work well when they eat. Your baby has the skill to close the jaw and lips on the spoon, so why not give her this practice?

The next method we will learn is "side-to-side" spoon-feeding. Sara Rosenfeld-Johnson and Lori Overland developed this spoon-feeding method.[252]

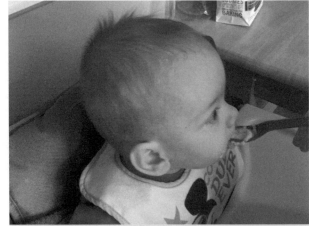

Photo 4.4: *Cannon (6.5 months) is making eye contact and removing food from the spoon with his lips during natural spoon-feeding with the small Maroon Spoon.*

1. Place one side of the spoon between your baby's lips, allowing her to take food off that side of the spoon using her lips. The edge of the spoon may lightly contact your baby's lip corners if you are using a spoon like the *small* Maroon Spoon.

2. Then turn your hand to allow your baby to take the food off of the other side of the spoon. This may be similar to the way you eat from a soup or ice cream spoon, and the method works best if you use a small spoon with a flat bowl.

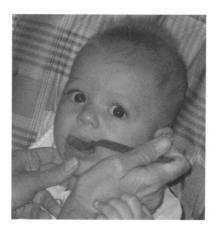
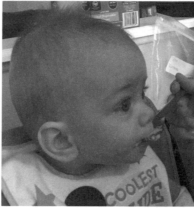

Photo 4.5: *Anthony (6 montwhs) and Cannon (6.5 months) work on "side-to-side" spoon feeding with a small Maroon Spoon (a method taught by Sara Rosenfeld-Johnson and Lori Overland). Anthony has a nice hand-mouth connection (his hand is on Diane's). Cannon is making good eye-contact with the feeder and sitting up well in his Keekaroo chair. Both Anthony and Cannon use their lips to remove the food from the spoon.*

Let your baby watch you eat food from a spoon. Babies are very tuned in to people's mouths. Eating is a social experience. Your baby will benefit by seeing you eat from the spoon. If you are eating something while your baby is eating, this will allow your baby some natural breaks during the meal. You can alternate giving your baby a bite of her food with taking a spoonful yourself.

Find a natural, easy pace when spoon-feeding your baby. This may depend on you and your baby's personalities. However, it's important not to feed your baby too rapidly, as this sets up a pattern she may carry throughout life. Some babies appear to want to spoon-feed very rapidly. This is probably related to the habit of drinking swallow after swallow, used during bottle or breastfeeding. You don't want your baby to develop a rapid spoon-feeding pattern, so you will teach her about pacing the meal.

Pacing a spoon-fed meal is important for several reasons. First, it allows your child to fully experience the shape, size, and texture of food in the mouth. As you know, digestion begins in the mouth as food is mixed with saliva. Second, the esophagus requires some time for the most efficient movement of food toward the stomach. Finally, the brain needs time to register the presence of food in the stomach, so your child will know when she is full. So, avoid feeding your baby when you feel rushed. Try turning on some soft back-ground music to relax you and your baby. And, talk to your baby as you feed her and have a meal together. See the Feeding and Related Development Checklist: Birth to 24 Months and Food and Liquid Introduction Checklist: Birth to 24 Months in Chapter 1 for further information.

How Does Your Baby Eat From a Spoon?

Place check marks in the columns next to the description matching what your baby is doing and things you may want to change.

WHAT YOU WANT MY BABY:	CHECK MARK	THINGS TO CHANGE MY BABY:	CHECK MARK
Eats from a spoon with a small, flat bowl that fits my baby's lips.	☐	Eats from a spoon that is too big or deep (such as a regular teaspoon).	☐
Watches me when I eat from a spoon.	☐	Does not have the opportunity to watch others eat from a spoon.	☐
Has a good rhythm and rate when eating from a spoon.	☐	Eats too fast or too slow.	☐
Eats a small and/or reasonable amount of food from the spoon.	☐	Eats large amounts from the spoon and loses a lot of food from the mouth.	☐
Closes her lips on the spoon, and waits for me to remove the spoon in a level manner.	☐	Allows me to scrape food off the upper lip or gum as I tip the spoon upward.	☐

An Important Note about Pouch Foods

Pouch foods are spoon foods, so please squeeze the food from the pouch into a bowl or directly onto the spoon when possible. Children who eat or suck directly from pouches without spoon-feeding and other feeding experiences are often delayed in their feeding skill development. Pouch foods only require sucking, and your baby got plenty of this practice from the breast or bottle.

Drinking from an Open Cup

Before you have your baby drink from an open cup, see how you drink from one. Try both regular thin liquid (like water) and a thicker liquid (such as tomato juice or a yogurt drink). Observe how you take liquid from an open cup and what you do once the liquid is in your mouth.

How Do You Drink from an Open Cup?

Place an answer next to each question. Take some sips and swallows from an open cup and observe the following.

QUESTIONS	YOUR ANSWERS
Is the cup placed just on your lower lip, or is it pressed or jammed into the corners of your mouth?	
What happens if you press the cup rim into the corners of your mouth? Can you really drink this way?	
Are your lips helping to keep you from spilling the liquid when you drink?	
Is your tongue under the cup when you drink? Hope not.	
What is the difference between taking one sip and drinking the liquid swallow after swallow?	
Does the tip of your tongue touch the indentation in the ridge behind your top front teeth to begin your swallow?	
Does the rest of your tongue cup and hold the liquid, and then move it back for the swallow?	

In a mature, sophisticated swallowing pattern, the tongue tip rises to an indentation in the ridge behind the top front teeth, the sides of the tongue rise cupping the liquid, and then the tongue squeezes the liquid back in a controlled, wavelike manner. The tongue has a slight bowl shape as the liquid is cupped in the center of the tongue. Some people either do not attain this mature pattern as children or they lose the ability to use this pattern (such as through stroke, brain injury, aging, etc.).

An unsophisticated swallowing pattern can lead to significant orthodontic concerns (such as overjet, overbite, and gaps between the teeth) and oral hygiene problems. This can also be associated with several speech errors (such as lisps, as well as persistent "r" and/or "l" distortions). These topics are covered in the book *Nobody Ever Told Me (or My Mother) That! Everything from Bottles and Breathing to Healthy Speech Development* by Diane Bahr.

How to Teach Your Baby Open Cup-Drinking

In my experience, drinking from an open cup is one of the easiest methods to use when feeding a baby. It has been used with babies born prematurely as well as babies having difficulty learning to drink from the breast or bottle. Open cup-drinking can be easier to teach than spoon-feeding. And, it is likely more similar to breastfeeding than bottle-feeding.[253][254][255][256][257] Five or 6 months of age is a good time to begin open cup-drinking. You can give your baby single sips of breast milk or formula from an open cup. This is a time when your child's lip, cheek, and tongue movements are becoming increasingly independent of her jaw movements.

Begin your baby's open cup-drinking process with a small but wide-mouthed open cup or a cut-out cup (also called a *nosey cup*). Medicine cups and clear plastic cocktail cups are frequently used as first cups because parents can easily see and control the movement of the liquid. Cut-out or nosey cups have often been used with children who have feeding difficulties. This means they are great cups for teaching the skill of drinking from a cup. The cut-out portion of the cup is placed on top, so

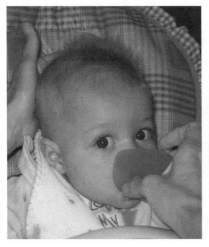 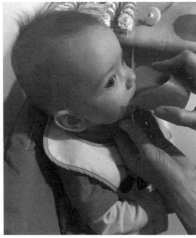

Photo 4.6: *Anthony (6 months) and Cannon (6.5 months) learn open cup-drinking from a small pink cut-out cup. Cannon brings his hands toward midline (the middle) which is likely step toward putting his hands on the cup.*

you can see the liquid in the cup and your child can drink without moving her head and neck too far back (hyperextension). Cut-out cups are available in a number of sizes. I use the small pink cut-out cup for my 6-month-old children when I teach open cup-drinking. See previous list of companies that carry feeding products for children that cannot be found in most stores (in the spoon-feeding section in this chapter).

Remember, when your child's head and neck are hyperextended, the airway is open (in a CPR position), and choking can occur more readily. When drinking from an open cup, your child's head needs to be in a neutral, aligned position, or your child's chin needs to be *slightly* tucked in with her ears just in front of her shoulders. It's also important you give your child a small and/or reasonable amount of liquid with each sip. You don't want to hear gulping or excessive coughing. The rim of the open cup (long side if using a cut-out cup) is placed on your child's lower lip. Teach your child to drink from the cup by giving one sip at a time. Be sure your child is not leaning into the cup and the cup is not pressed or jammed into the corners of her lips. It's almost impossible to drink this way. Hold the cup during this process but encourage your child over time to place her hands on the sides of the cup. This is a nice hand-mouth activity for your child as hands and mouths are meant to work together.

I usually place a thickened liquid into the open cup when I teach the skill of drinking from an open cup. This allows the parent to control the flow of the liquid. It also allows the child to receive greater sensory information from the liquid as well. First liquids could include formula or breast milk thickened slightly with baby cereal if you begin cup-drinking at 6 months. Also, stage-one baby food fruits and sweet vegetables (such as carrots or squash) can be thinned with water and served from an open cup. When you and your child are comfortable with the single-sip drinking process, you can begin using regular thin liquids (such as formula, breast milk, and water), unless you already introduced formula and breast milk from an open cup prior to 6 months of age.

When your child is taking single sips from an open cup, be sure the cup rim is placed on her lower lip and your child's tongue is *not* under the cup. Your child's tongue may occasionally slip under the cup because of the drinking pattern she used previously with the bottle and/or breast. I have found it is better to reposition the open cup on the child's lower lip when giving her single sips, so poor cup-drinking habits are not established. However, you may notice your child biting on the cup rim to stabilize her jaw. This keeps her jaw still while she learns to use her lips, cheeks, and tongue independently from her jaw. This can be typical until 18+ months of age. In fact, many adults gently rest the cup rim against their teeth when drinking swallow after swallow from an open cup.

After your child has become proficient at taking single sips from an open cup, she will begin taking longer drinks from the open cup by using more than one swallow. This develops between 6 and 12 months of age as your child's breathing and swallowing coordination is maturing. Your child will probably be drinking regular thin liquids (such as formula, breast milk, and water) at this time. However, if your child is having difficulty learning to swallow consecutively (swallow after swallow), you may want to use a slightly thickened liquid until she becomes comfortable with this process.

Assist your child by holding the open cup with her as she learns to consecutively swallow the liquid. Your child will begin by taking 2 or 3 consecutive swallows of liquid at one time. Her head should be in a neutral position (aligned with the body), and her chin may be slightly tucked in. Be sure she is not leaning into the cup. Again, you don't want to hear gulping or excessive coughing. Be sure you are giving her a reasonable amount of liquid during this process (not too much). See the Feeding and Related Development Checklist: Birth to 24 Months in Chapter 1 for further information.

You may have heard about the controversy surrounding the use of spouted or sippy cups. These cups seem to promote the use of unsophisticated drinking and swallowing patterns. Children appear to drink from sippy cups like they drink from bottles. The pattern your child uses when drinking from a bottle is different than the pattern she uses in the more mature process of drinking from an open cup. Drinking from an open cup, like spoon-feeding, involves greater lip and cheek activity, as well as more independent jaw, lip, cheek, and tongue movements than those used in bottle drinking. Sippy cups can impede your child's development of appropriate drinking and swallowing skills because they seem to encourage her to maintain old patterns used with drinking from a bottle.

This becomes a particular concern when the tip of the tongue should be learning to elevate or rise during the development of the mature swallowing pattern (around 11 to 12 months of age). The tongue tip cannot rise to the alveolar ridge behind the top front teeth for the mature swallow when the spout of the sippy cup is placed into the mouth. The spout is in the way. In some children, you can see the whole jaw moving front and back as they drink from a sippy cup. This is not the pattern we want to see during cup-drinking. We want to see slight up-down jaw movement which began with proper breastfeeding.

The potential problems caused by sippy cup use cannot be overstated. These include the interruption of the development of the mature swallowing pattern and liquid tending to remain in the mouth rather than being swallowed (which can lead to tooth decay). Dentists and therapists have long been concerned about the use of spouted cups for these reasons. Although they may be convenient, sippy cups should be avoided when possible.[258][259][260][261]

There are actually a number of other spill-proof or spill-resistant cup options such as cups with recessed lids and straws from which your child can be taught to properly drink by 12 months of age. A cup with a recessed lid has a lip similar to an open cup and is used like one. However, the lid helps the child avoid spilling the liquid. These cups come with and without handles. See previous list of companies that carry feeding products for children that cannot be found in most stores (in the spoon-feeding section in this chapter).

How Does Your Baby Drink From an Open Cup?

Place check marks in the columns next to the description that matches what your baby is doing and things you may want to change.

WHAT YOU WANT MY BABY:	CHECK MARK	THINGS TO CHANGE MY BABY:	CHECK MARK
Drinks from an open cup that fits her mouth.	☐	Drinks from a cup that is too big or too small.	☐
Allows the open cup to be placed just on her bottom lip.	☐	Leans into the cup with lip corners pressed or jammed against the cup or has her tongue under the cup.	☐
Takes one small sip of thickened liquid (such as stage one baby food thinned with water) at a time at 6 months.	☐	Gulps or chokes on liquid.	☐
Takes one small sip of thin liquid at a time when ready.	☐	Gulps or chokes on liquid.	☐
Drinks swallow after swallow in a coordinated manner between 6 and 12 months.	☐	Has a lot of jaw movement and/or leans into cup when trying to take swallow after swallow.	☐

Drinking from a Straw

Before you introduce your baby to straw-drinking, observe how you drink liquid from a straw. What do you do once the liquid is in your mouth?

How Do You Drink From a Straw?

Place an answer next to each question. Take some sips and swallows from a straw and observe the following.

QUESTIONS	YOUR ANSWERS
Is the straw placed far into your mouth onto your tongue, or is it just on your lips? If you place the straw far into your mouth onto your tongue, then you are using an unsophisticated swallowing pattern. See what it is like to just place the straw on your lips.	

QUESTIONS	YOUR ANSWERS
Do you place the straw in the center of your lips or to the side? If you place the straw to the side, you may have a stronger side. This may also be related to your hand dominance (right-handed or left-handed). See what it is like to place the straw in the center of your lips.	
If you place the straw just onto your lips (not onto your tongue) to drink, do you pull your tongue back slightly? Can your tongue tip rise to the ridge behind your top front teeth to start the swallow?	
Can you drink swallow after swallow from the straw?	
Can you feel the muscles in your abdomen (just below your belly button) and diaphragm (at the bottom of your ribcage) working? Place your hands on these areas as you suck through the straw to feel your muscles working. These are the same muscles you use in breathing.	

How To Teach Your Baby to Drink from a Straw

In addition to spoon-feeding and open cup-drinking, straw-drinking can be taught around 6 months of age using a squeezable bottle with a straw. These bottles are available from TalkTools, ARK Therapeutic, and others. See previous list of companies that carry feeding products for children that cannot be found in most stores (in the spoon-feeding section in this chapter).

You can easily *make a squeezable bottle with a straw*. Here are the directions:

1. Use a bottle that is approved to contain food (such as a squeezable honey-bear, sauce, or cake decorating bottle). While glue and hair color bottles look similar, they are not meant to hold food or consumable liquid, so *do not use them.*

2. Once you choose your bottle, make a straw from a piece of plumbing or refrigerator tubing that fits the opening of the squeezable bottle (approximately ¼ of an inch in diameter and long enough to reach the bottom of the bottle). Plumbing and refrigerator tubing is designed to carry water, so it's considered safe to use as a straw. Place the plumbing tubing through the top of the bottle by cutting the bottle top to fit the tubing in a snug manner. You can purchase

plumbing or refrigerator tubing from a hardware store. Please *do not use* aquarium tubing as it may contain toxins.

Here are the directions for *teaching your child how to drink from a squeezable bottle with a straw*, beginning around 6 months of age.

1. Place a thickened liquid into the squeezable straw bottle. A thickened liquid will provide you with improved control and will give your child increased sensory information while learning this new skill. As previously mentioned with open cup-drinking, thickened liquids can include formula or breast milk thickened with baby cereal or appropriate stage-one baby foods thinned with water. Some babies can learn to drink from a straw using non-thickened breast milk or formula.

2. If you are teaching straw-drinking to an older child (over 12 months), you can use a yogurt drink or fruit nectar. Check with your child's pediatrician about when you can introduce these drinks.

3. Once your thickened liquid is placed into your squeezable bottle, insert the straw and seal the bottle (top screws on). Softly squeeze the thickened liquid so it reaches the top of the straw. Practice this several times before you present it to your baby. You do not want to accidentally squirt your baby in the face with the liquid.

4. After you become skilled in squeezing the liquid to the top of the straw, place the end of the straw on the center of your child's lower lip. About ¼ inch of the straw should be placed on your child's lip. The straw should not extend into your child's mouth. Your baby's tongue should not be under the straw because this is the pattern your child already uses on a bottle (if he or she drinks from a bottle). We want to teach your child something new with straw-drinking.

5. Once you place the straw on the center of your baby's lower lip, wait for her to close her lips around the straw. Some children learn this very quickly because they already know how to close their lips on a bottle nipple. Allow your baby to take one sip from the straw and remove the straw from her mouth. You can repeatedly place the straw on your baby's lips for more single sips. Most babies can easily learn to take sips this way. However, if your baby has difficulty rounding her lips on the straw you can provide some careful, gentle cheek support (as discussed in Chapter 3) to help her learn to round her lips. Remember, cheeks help activate lips.

6. Some babies may need a taste of the liquid to get them started or interested. If you squeeze the bottle just a little more, you can give your baby a small taste. However, it's very important you don't squirt a large amount of liquid into your baby's mouth, as this can overwhelm your baby. We don't want to place more liquid into your child's mouth than she can handle.

7. After your child has learned to take single sips from the straw, she will learn to take consecutive sips and swallows on her own (you will no longer need to squeeze the bottle). Many babies learn

this very quickly, but some take more time. Consecutive swallowing (taking swallow after swallow) is a more complex task than taking single sips. However, your baby already does this with breastfeeding and/or bottle-feeding. Your child will learn to take consecutive sips and swallows from a straw with a little consistent practice. Just be patient and hold the straw bottle at your child's lips during this process.

8. Again, try not to let the straw slip too far into your baby's mouth, or your baby will begin drinking from the straw in a similar way as a child drinks from a bottle. Always check to be sure the straw is placed just on your child's lips, so the lips and cheeks can do the work instead of the tongue.

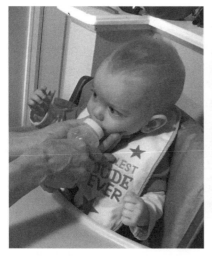
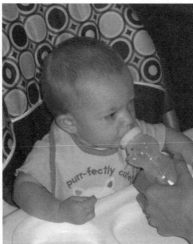

Photo 4.7: *Cannon (6.5 months) is learning straw-drinking with the straw bear and gentle jaw and cheek support. Rylee (7.5 months) is learning straw-drinking with the straw bear without jaw support. The straw is placed on the child's lips only (not into the mouth) during this process.*

Note: There is a one-way straw mechanism that can be attached to the bottom of a straw. This will keep the liquid from going back down the straw and into the bottle. See previous list of companies that carry feeding products for children that cannot be found in most stores (in the spoon-feeding section in this chapter).

Once your child has learned to drink from the squeezable straw bottle, he or she can begin using a cup with a straw. This can be a cup with a flip-up straw or a cup with a hole for a regular straw (such as the First Years Take & Toss straw cup). I have worked with many children who were ready to drink from a cup with a regular straw between 9 and 12 months of age. You will place regular thin liquids into the cup when your child is ready (when he can drink thin liquids on his own from the straw without excessive coughing or choking).

One problem with some cups with flip-up straws is they are labeled for older children (such as 2 years and up). However, I have taught many 12-month-old children to drink from these cups. Another problem with most flip-up straws is they are too long and need to be shortened. You can cut the straw or place a bumper on the straw to help your child with the process *if you can do this safely* (we don't want loose parts that can become a choking hazard). Remember, appropriate straw use requires your child to place the straw *only on his lips* (not into the mouth and onto the tongue).

Lip bumpers can be made by drilling a straw-size hole through a cork. The cork then fits snuggly on the straw and only allows ¼ inch of the straw to sit on your child's lips. You want a safe device to keep the straw from going into your child's mouth onto his tongue. You do not want a device that will break into pieces and become a choking hazard. TalkTools and ARK Therapeutic carry ready-made lip bumpers for straws. TalkTools also has a formalized straw program for older children. These companies are found in a previous list of companies that carry feeding equipment not typically found in stores (in the spoon-feeding section in this chapter).

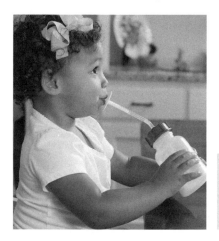

Now, let's summarize why you would want to begin teaching the skill of straw-drinking to your baby around 6 months of age. First of all, straw-drinking is a skill your baby can use throughout life. Also, drinking from open- and recessed-lid cups as well as straws can replace spouted or sippy cup use. Remember, sippy cups encourage your child to use an unsophisticated swallowing pattern similar to the one used on a baby bottle.

Photo 4.8: *ARK Therapeutic provides (with permission) the photo of a child using an ARK Cip-Kup with an ARK Lip Blok Mouthpiece. These mouthpieces are available in different lengths, so the child can eventually just place the straw on the lips and not into the mouth (www.ARKTherapeutic.com).*

The proper technique for drinking from a straw, like drinking from an open cup, allows your child to lift his tongue tip to the ridge behind the top front teeth to start the mature swallow. Sippy cups impede this process because the spout gets in the way of the tongue-tip lifting. The mature swallowing pattern is important for clearing the mouth of food and liquid. Individuals who do not develop this pattern tend to have food or liquid remaining in the mouth after swallowing. This can lead to difficulties with oral hygiene.

Also, individuals who do not develop a mature swallowing pattern tend to use other unsophisticated oral movement patterns (such as not chewing food well and swallowing food whole which can lead to poor digestion and metabolism of nutrients in food). When someone uses an unsophisticated swallowing pattern, the tongue tends to move with the jaw. When the tongue, jaw, lips, and cheeks do not learn to work independently of one another, food and liquid are generally not managed well or efficiently.

The tongue tip rising to the ridge behind the top front teeth is also an important movement for the speech sounds "t," "d," "n," and "l." Try making these sounds and see where your tongue goes. While swallowing and speech require different movement patterns or sequences in your child's brain, the movements are similar in terms of placement and direction. More information on speech development and mature swallowing can be found in the book *Nobody Ever Told Me (or My Mother) That! Everything from Bottles and Breathing to Healthy Speech Development* by Diane Bahr.

How Does Your Baby Drink From a Straw?

Place check marks in the columns next to the description matching what your baby is doing and things you may want to change.

WHAT YOU WANT MY BABY:	CHECK MARK	THINGS TO CHANGE MY BABY:	CHECK MARK
Drinks from a straw placed just on the lips.	☐	Drinks from a straw placed far into the mouth onto the tongue.	☐
Drinks from a straw placed in the center of the lips.	☐	Drinks from a straw placed to one side of the lips.	☐
Can take one sip at a time from a straw, with the straw placed just on the lips.	☐	Places the straw deeply into the mouth like a baby bottle nipple.	☐
Can drink swallow after swallow from a straw placed just on the lips.	☐	Places the straw far into the mouth to drink swallow after swallow.	☐

Taking Bites and Chewing Safe, Appropriate Foods

Before you give your baby food to bite and chew, see how you accomplish these processes. Get a soft cookie (such as an arrowroot, butter, or Lorna Doone cookie). Observe how you take bites of the cookie and what you do with the cookie after you take the bite.

How Do You Take Bites and Chew Food?

Place an answer next to each question. Take some bites of a soft cookie or cracker and observe the following.

QUESTIONS	YOUR ANSWERS
Do you take bites of the cookie with your front teeth or those toward the side? If you take bites toward the side, this may have to do with the hand you use to feed yourself or your dentition (how your teeth meet).	

QUESTIONS	YOUR ANSWERS
How large of a bite do you take? Hopefully, it's not too large.	
Does the tip of your tongue move this bite of cookie to your back molars for chewing?	
After chewing, does the tip of your tongue help collect the chewed cookie and bring it back to the center of your tongue for the swallow?	
Does the tip of your tongue then lift to the bump or ridge behind your top front teeth to start the swallow? If not, you may be using an unsophisticated swallowing pattern. Many adults have never developed a fully mature swallowing pattern. This ultimately can lead to oral hygiene and dental concerns.	

How to Teach Your Baby to Safely Take Bites of Food and Chew Properly

At 6 months of age, babies are ready to begin taking bites of soft cookies and learning to chew them. Your baby can also begin to have some lumps to chew in his baby food. This will automatically happen if you make your own baby food with a food blender, grinder, mill, or processor. When you are ready to give your baby safe foods for biting and chewing, consider the size of your baby's jaw. Soft, non-wheat cookies and biscuits, such as the arrowroot cookies and Baby Mum-Mum rice biscuits, are a good place to start because they melt down easily in your baby's mouth. This decreases the risk of choking. Some baby cookies and toast (such as teething biscuits and zwieback toast) are too large for the mouth of a 6-month-old child, and they are not considered soft cookies.

It's also important to give your baby cookies and biscuits made for babies. You don't want to give your baby cookies or crackers containing preservatives or foods that are not safe for babies. While many people think Cheerios are a safe first food for babies, they have a rather crunchy, hard texture. I don't feel comfortable giving these to a child until he has developed some skill with chewing. When you introduce a soft cookie or biscuit to your baby, hold it to his lips. Allow him to hold the cookie with you if possible. He may use both hands. Don't forget the hands and the mouth are meant to work together. Humans seem to be internally programmed to do this.

Let your baby explore the safe, soft cookie or biscuit with his lips and gums. Your baby has an innate biting response that will help him or her begin biting on the soft cookie or biscuit when it touches and/or presses against his gums. He will bite, bite, bite on the cookie or biscuit to soften it, and a piece will break off. The first time this occurs, your baby may appear surprised or make a funny face. It's important for you to monitor the size of the bite your baby takes. However, a soft baby cookie or biscuit will usually soften and break down easily in the mouth.

Some parents are very concerned about giving their babies solid foods because they are afraid of choking. If soft, safe, solid foods are introduced appropriately, your baby will gain the skills he needs at the appropriate time. Some parents think a baby cannot chew because he does not have teeth. However, teeth emerge as the gums are stimulated. Introducing safe and appropriate food textures for biting and chewing when your child is ready for them will help teeth develop. See Food and Liquid Introduction Checklist: Birth to 24 Months in Chapter 1.

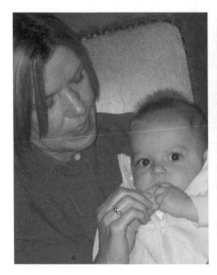 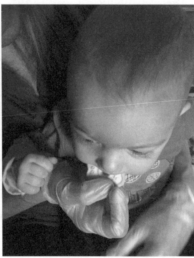

Photo 4.9: *Anthony (6 months) and Cannon (6.5 months) have their first arrowroot cookie with Diane. Anthony has his hand on the cookie, and Cannon has his hand on Diane's hand. Both boys have good hand-mouth connections.*

Taking bites and chewing is crucial for jaw development and independent tongue, lip, cheek, and jaw movement used in mature eating and drinking skills. This helps your child maintain adequate jaw strength as the jaw grows. The muscles of the jaw need appropriate strength, and they readjust constantly as the jawbones grows. The lower jawbone is a heavy bone, and the muscle function of the jaw needs to keep up with the growth of this bone and the upper jawbone. See jaw development diagrams from Dr. David C. Page, Sr. in Chapter 2.

Lips and cheeks work together because cheeks help to activate lips. The lips and cheeks need to move independently from the jaw to assist in getting, keeping, and managing food and/or liquid in the mouth. The tongue becomes increasingly skilled over time in the placement and collection of food and liquid within the mouth. The cheeks also move inward to help establish appropriate intraoral pressure during the mature swallow.

By 11 to 12 months of age, your baby will begin to demonstrate a mature oral swallow if his tongue tip is not blocked by a nipple, spout, or too much food in the mouth. In the mature oral swallow, the tongue tip begins the swallow by touching or contacting the ridge or bump behind the top front teeth. The food or liquid is collected in the center of the tongue and then moved back by a wavelike motion toward the throat for the swallow. See Feeding and Related Development Checklist: Birth to 24 Months in Chapter 1 for detailed information.

If you are afraid to introduce foods for your baby to bite or chew, use a safety net. A safe feeder allows you to place bite-sized pieces of food into a silicon or mesh receptacle for chewing. Your baby can then chew on the foods in the silicon or mesh container while holding onto a handle. As the food breaks down, it will come through the mesh or holes in the silicon in very small pieces for manipulation and swallowing. There are a number of safe feeders on the market. However, many mesh or silicon receptacles of safe feeders are much too large. This allows large pieces of food to be placed into the netting or pouch, which makes it difficult for your baby to bite and chew on food using all gum surfaces (front, side, and back). Taking bites of food occurs in the front of the mouth. Over time, the tongue learns to follow and place food in the back-gum area, and chewing food occurs where the molars will eventually emerge. When you place food into a safe feeder, be sure you only place a small, baby-bite-sized piece of food into the receptacle, so your baby can move this throughout the mouth and to the back molar areas. The bite-sized piece of food needs to fit your baby's mouth, so it is much smaller than a bite you would take. An example of an appropriate safe feeder is the *small* KidsMe feeder.

Therapists have also used cheesecloth to create little pouches to hold food for chewing. Cheesecloth can often be purchased in grocery stores. Unwrap and cut a section of cheesecloth (which is packaged in a triple thickness). Place a baby-bite-sized piece of food into the center of the cheesecloth and close the cheesecloth around it. Twist the cheesecloth into a sack or pouch, *so you can hold onto it* without losing the food while your baby chews on the food in the cheesecloth. Unlike the safe feeder, you will need to hold the cheesecloth as your baby chews. If your baby places his hands on your hands, this again represents the very natural hand-mouth connection.

Now, here is an activity you can do with baby-bite-sized pieces of food wrapped in cheesecloth or placed into an appropriately sized safe feeder.

1. Place the baby-bite-sized piece of food onto your baby's gums in the cheesecloth or safe feeder.

2. Let your baby hold the cheesecloth or safe feeder with you.

3. Press gently but firmly into the bottom or top gum with the food in the cheesecloth or feeder to remind your baby to begin chewing.

4. Work the bite-sized piece of food in the cheesecloth or safe feeder from the front of your baby's mouth to the back where the molars will eventually emerge. Your baby will be taking little bites

all along the way, as the food in the cheesecloth or safe feeder is worked toward the molar areas. You will also see your baby's tongue move toward the feeder.

5. You can let your baby chew food naturally at one back molar area and then the other.

6. You can encourage your baby to chew food placed in the cheesecloth or safe feeder 12 to 15 times (or up to 20 to 25 times) at each back molar area, alternating sides. However, if your baby only wants to chew 6 times on a side, that is fine. Maybe he will want to chew 7 times during his next opportunity. Follow his lead.

7. You can alternate chewing sides 2 more times (for 3 sets total) if your baby is interested and having fun. However, be sensitive to your baby's interest level, abilities, and communication. If your baby becomes fatigued (if his chewing begins to feel weak) or disorganized (if he loses his chewing rhythm), stop and move to the other side, or take a break.

8. While your child may demonstrate a preferred side of the mouth for chewing, try to have him chew the same number of times on each side. This will help balance the movements of the jaw. Chewing is the *best possible exercise* for the jaw. It helps the jaw grow properly. And, if the jaw is doing what it needs to do, then the cheeks, lips, and tongue can do what they need to do provided your baby does not have a restriction (such as tongue tie).

As food moves through the safe feeder or cheesecloth, replace it with another baby-bite-sized piece of food. If you are using a safe feeder or food in cheesecloth, you can introduce foods other than the soft baby cookies or biscuits we discussed earlier. You can place baby bite-sized pieces of cooled, soft, steamed vegetables (such as carrots or squash) or cooled, parboiled fruit without skin (such as apples, peaches, or pears) into the safe feeder or cheesecloth. As your child's abilities to take bites and chew foods become more sophisticated, you can begin to give him these and other foods without the cheesecloth or safe feeder. See Food and Liquid Introduction Checklist: Birth to 24 Months in Chapter 1.

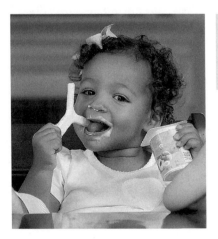

Photo 4.10: *ARK Therapeutic provides (with permission) the photo of a child using an ARK Y-Chew to do some good chewing at the back molar area while adding the yummy taste of yogurt to the process. What fun! (www.ARKTherapeutic.com).*

This activity is excellent exercise for your baby's jaw muscles. It helps your baby develop graded jaw movement (the ability to move the jaw as needed for the particular activity) and independent movement of the cheeks, lips, and tongue from the jaw. These skills are important in the development of mature eating and drinking skills. As your baby begins to chew on foods and appropriate toys at 6 months of age, chewing can begin to replace sucking and suckling for calming. See section on Appropriate Mouth Items and Toys in this chapter. This is the time when you can begin to wean your baby from the pacifier if he is using one. Specific information on pacifier weaning can be found in the book *Nobody Ever Told Me (or My Mother) That! Everything from Bottles and Breathing to Healthy Speech Development* by Diane Bahr.

How Does Your Baby Take Bites and Chew Foods?

Place check marks in the columns next to the description matching what your baby is doing and things you may want to change.

WHAT YOU WANT My 6- to 7-month-old baby:	CHECK MARK	THINGS TO CHANGE My 6- to 7-month-old baby:	CHECK MARK
Takes little phasic bites (a rhythmic bite, bite, bite) of a soft cookie held by baby and me at the front of his mouth.	☐	Only sucks on the soft cookie.	☐
Chews on small lumps of food even without teeth.	☐	Only sucks or does not eat food with lumps.	☐
Moves his tongue toward food in the side of the mouth.	☐	Doesn't move his tongue toward food in the side of the mouth.	☐

Weaning from Bottle and Breast

This process starts when your baby begins to drink from open cups and straws around 6 months of age. You will initially place breast milk and/or formula into these cups as your child learns to use them until your child's pediatrician tells you to offer other liquids (such as water usually around 6 months). You will use these cups more frequently as your child becomes skilled in their use. By 12 to 15 months of age, most of your child's liquid will be given by open cup, recessed-lid cup, or straw.

As your child learns to drink from an open cup, recessed-lid cup, and straw, praise him. Be sure to provide your baby with suitable mouth activities to appropriately replace the stimulation he received from the bottle and/or breast. Spoon-feeding, open cup-, recessed-lid cup-, straw-drinking, taking bites of food and chewing, as well as biting and chewing on appropriate mouth toys will help to fulfill this need. See Appropriate Mouth Items and Toys in this chapter. Every child is unique, so the weaning process is different for each child. Do not stress yourself or your child during this progression. Go slowly. Replace bottle-feeding and/or breastfeeding throughout the day as you and your child are ready. You have 6 to 9 months for bottle weaning (from the time your child is 6 months of age until 12 to 15 months).

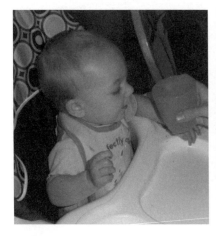

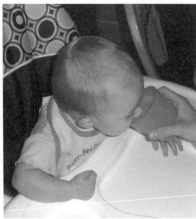

Photo 4.11: *Rylee (7.5 months) learns to drink from a regular open cup. She gets her mouth ready and then moves in toward the cup, but the cup is only placed on her lips (not pressed into her lip corners).*

If your child's pediatrician is in agreement, you can add water to formula or breast milk in the bottle during the weaning process and present the undiluted formula or breast milk in a cup. This way your child is rewarded with the full taste of the formula or breast milk while drinking from the cup.[262]

Note: It's very important to work closely with your child's pediatrician on this process to ensure your child is getting proper nutrition and hydration.

By 12 to 15 months of age, your child will take the bottle or breast primarily around bedtime. All other liquid will be taken from an open cup, a cup with a recessed lid, or a straw. During the weaning process, we want your baby to breastfeed or bottle-feed before bed, *not in bed*. Remember, you have not allowed your baby to take a bottle lying down because of the related risk of ear problems. If your baby has reflux or a history of reflux, you may want to give your child the bottle or breast before bath and reading time. This will allow him to be upright for a while before sleep. If you have experienced reflux, you know it's worse at night when you eat or drink just before lying down in bed.

If your child is still seeking comfort to fall asleep at night, you can provide him with safe mouth toys. He can appropriately mouth or chew on these prior to sleep. See section on Appropriate Mouth Items and Toys in this chapter. You have hopefully already weaned your child from the pacifier between 6 and 10 months if your baby used a pacifier. See guidelines for pacifier weaning in the book *Nobody Ever Told Me (or My Mother) That! Everything from Bottles and Breathing to Healthy Speech Development* by Diane Bahr.

When weaning your child from the bottle or breast, you can start to skip some evening feedings by replacing them with a snack before bedtime. This can include a drink from an open cup, a cup with a recessed lid, or a straw, as well as some food. Do this when your child is in good mood and not too tired. Remember, children often derive comfort from sucking at the breast or on the bottle. While you read a story and look at books with your child after snack and bath time, allow him to chew on and mouth appropriate mouth toys. This will help to satisfy your child's need for oral stimulation and can improve attention, focus, and concentration. As adults, we often chew gum for this purpose,

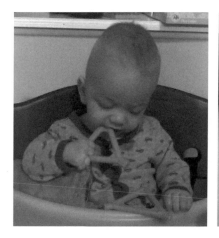
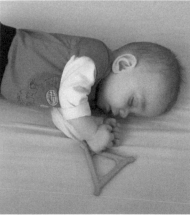

Photo 4.12: *After finishing his lunch, Cannon (6.5 months) wonders which mouth toy to choose for his nap (on left). He decided on the green Beckman Tri-Chew for his nap instead of sucking his thumb (on right).*

as well as to keep gastroesophageal reflux under control. See information on the use of appropriate mouth toys in the book *Nobody Ever Told Me (or My Mother) That! Everything from Bottles and Breathing to Healthy Speech Development* by Diane Bahr. A listing of appropriate mouth toys by age is found in the next section.

If your child asks for the breast or bottle on an evening where you have replaced a feeding with a snack and drink, explain to him that he is getting to be a big boy. Reassure and praise him by saying how proud and happy you are. As you go through this process, be patient and supportive of yourself and your child. Offer your child choices of snacks, drinks, and mouth toys (For example, "Do you want a cookie or cracker? Do you want milk or water? Do you want a Chewy Tube or Y-Chew?"). You can offer one preferred item and one that is less preferred to increase your child's incentive to choose. This helps him become part of the process and makes life easier for both of you.

Twelve to 15 months of age is a good time to finish weaning your child from the bottle to help assist good mouth development. You may continue breastfeeding for 2 years or beyond. You have been giving your child experiences with the open cup, recessed-lid cup, and straw cup since 6 months of age. These are important skills he will use throughout life. Your child *never* needs to use a sippy cup. The problem with sippy cup use at 11 to 15 months of age and beyond is that it is used like a bottle. If a straw is used improperly (placed too far into the mouth), it is also used like a bottle. However, you have learned about proper cup and straw use in this chapter.

Congratulations! You are ready to wean your child from the breast and/or bottle. You are also helping your child develop the mature swallowing pattern he will use throughout life.

Weaning From Breast or Bottle Checklist

Place check marks in the column next to the description matching what you and your child are doing during the weaning process.

4 TO 6 MONTHS	CHECK MARK
Begin having your baby take sips from an open cup using formula or breast milk.	☐
Provide other appropriate mouth activities for your baby. See next section.	☐
6 TO 9 MONTHS	
Continue having your baby drink from an open cup by using appropriately thickened or regular liquid (such as breast milk, formula, or water).	☐
Begin teaching your baby to drink from a straw by using a specially made, squeezable bottle with thickened liquids (such as formula or breast milk thickened with baby cereal or stage one baby food thinned with water).	☐
Provide other appropriate mouth activities for your baby. See next section.	☐
9 TO 12 MONTHS	
Provide drinks (formula, breast milk, water) throughout the day with an open cup, straw, and/or cup with a recessed lid.	☐
Provide other appropriate mouth activities for your baby. See next section.	☐
12 TO 15 MONTHS	
Only give your baby the bottle at nighttime before bed, with the child sitting upright (can dilute milk in bottle with water if pediatrician says OK); may continue breastfeeding.	☐
Give remaining liquid (milk, water, very diluted fruit or vegetable juice) throughout the day from an open cup, a cup with a recessed lid, or straw (your child should be able to drink from a straw on his or her own).	☐

12 TO 15 MONTHS continued	
You may also want to give your child a cup with handles.	☐
Provide other appropriate mouth activities for your child. See next section.	☐
15 TO 18 MONTHS	
Your child is weaned from the bottle and is drinking from an open cup, a cup with a recessed lid, or straw; may continue some breastfeeding.	☐
Provide other appropriate mouth activities for your baby. See next section.	☐

Appropriate Mouth Items and Toys

The mouth items and toys in this section are recommended as your child grows. Most of these can be ordered from ARK Therapeutic or TalkTools as they are not available in stores. However, if you follow the guidelines in Chapters 4 and 5 of *Nobody Ever Told Me (or My Mother) That! Everything from Bottles and Breathing to Healthy Speech Development* by Diane Bahr, you can find some appropriate mouth toys in regular stores.

It's crucial to provide safe, appropriate mouth items and toys that fit your child's mouth for generalized and discriminative mouthing. Those that are too large or too difficult will not give your child the desired result. Generalized mouthing is where your baby sucks, mouths, and bites on safe

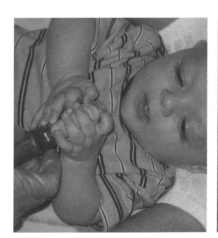
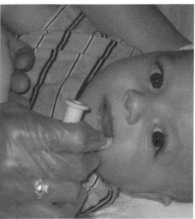

Photo 4.13: *Anthony (4 months) is getting ready to mouth a toy in a generalized manner at the front of his mouth (on left). However, he will chew on a yellow Chewy Tube with assistance (on right).*

items near the front of his mouth. Discriminative mouthing is where your child explores, bites on, and chews on items throughout his mouth. Good oral discrimination is needed for eating, drinking, and speaking.

The mouth items and toys in the chart are good for generalized mouthing (birth to 5 or 6 months), discriminative mouthing (5 to 6 months and beyond), teething, and exploration throughout the mouth. It's important your baby and toddler bite and chew on appropriate toys using the front, side, and back gum surfaces as part of teething. Mouth toy exploration and chewing activities can be done as you look at books or view videos together. Remember, chewing can help increase attention, focus, and concentration in any age individual. Do you ever chew gum?

Here are some resources to help you with the appropriate use of mouth toys:

- ChewyTubes, the work of Mary Shiavoni (chewytubes.com)

- *Nobody Ever Told Me (or My Mother) That! Everything from Bottles and Breathing to Healthy Speech Development by Diane Bahr* [263]

- *Tips & Techniques Exercise Book for the Grabber Family* by Debra Lowsky [264]

- *M.O.R.E.: Integrating the Mouth with Sensory and Postural Functions* by Patricia Oetter, Eileen Richter, and Shiela Frick [265]

- *OPT (Oral Placement Therapy) for Speech Clarity and Feeding* by Sara Rosenfeld-Johnson [266]

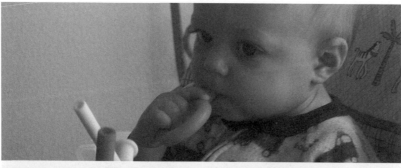

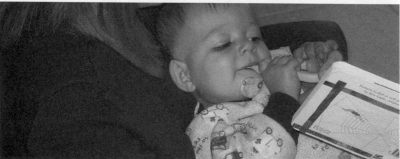

Photo 4.14: *Anthony (12 months) chooses to chew on the orange Chewy Q (on the top). And then, he chooses to look at a book while chewing on the green ARK Grabber (on the bottom).*

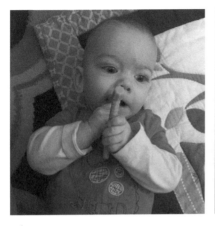

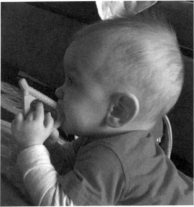

Photo 4.15: *Cannon (6.5 months) is chewing on and discriminatively mouthing his Beckman Tri-Chews. Hands and mouths work together in utero and hopefully throughout life. Babies go through periods of generalized mouthing (birth to 5 months) and discriminative mouthing (5 to 9 months and beyond).*

Some Recommended Mouthing Items or Toys by Age

Use this chart to make notes regarding your child's preferred mouthing items or toys. The toys from ARK Therapeutic and ChewyTubes are made in the United States of America from approved materials. TalkTools and ARK Therapeutic sell many of these. See companies that carry feeding products for children that cannot be found in most stores (in the spoon-feeding section in this chapter).

BIRTH TO 3 MONTHS (GENERALIZED MOUTHING)

- Baby's own hand and fingers, parent's finger.

Notes:

3 TO 4 MONTHS (GENERALIZED MOUTHING)

- Debra Beckman's Tri-Chews by ARK
- ARK's Baby Grabbers or Baby Guitars
- Chewy and Knobby Q's by ChewyTubes
- (All of the above used with parent help and supervision)

Notes:

5 TO 9 MONTHS (DISCRIMINATIVE MOUTHING)

- Chewy and Knobby Q's by ChewyTubes
- Yellow Chewy Tube (7+ months)
- Debra Beckman's Tri-Chews by ARK
- ARK's Baby Grabber, Soft Grabbers, or Baby Guitars

- Other appropriately sized mouth toys or items approved for use in the mouth
- (All of the above used with parent supervision)

Notes:

9 TO 12 MONTHS (BEGINNING TRUE MOUTH PLAY)

- Yellow and Red Chewy Tubes
- P's and Q's or Super Chews by ChewyTubes
- ARK's Grabbers, Y-Chews, or Guitars
- Baby Horns and Bubbles (with parent activation, demonstration, and presentation to the child for use)

- Other appropriately sized toys or items approved for use in the mouth
- (All of the above used with parent supervision)

Notes:

12 TO 18 MONTHS (TRUE MOUTH PLAY)

- Yellow and Red Chewy Tubes
- Knobby Tubes
- P's and Q's or Super Chews by Chewy Tubes
- ARK's Grabbers, Y-Chews, or Guitars

- Horns and Bubbles (with parent activation, demonstration, and presentation to child for use)
- Other appropriately sized toys or items approved for use in the mouth
- (All of the above used with parent supervision)

Notes:

18 TO 24 MONTHS (TRUE MOUTH PLAY)

- Yellow and Red Chewy Tubes
- Knobby Tubes
- P's and Q's or Super Chews by ChewyTubes
- ARK's Grabbers, Y-Chews, or Guitars

- Horns and Bubbles (with parent activation, demonstration, and presentation to child for use)
- Other appropriately sized toys or items approved for use in the mouth
- (All of the above used with parent supervision)

Notes:

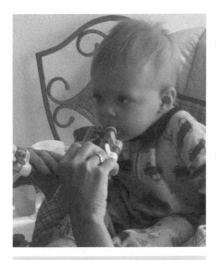

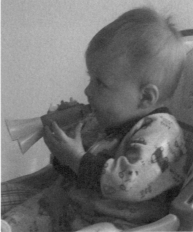

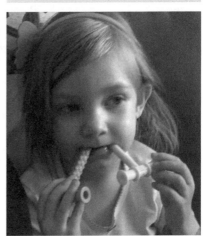

Photo 4.16: *Anthony (12 months) participates in horn play with wonderful eye contact. Horn play encourages controlled breathing.*

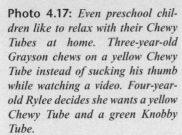

Photo 4.17: *Even preschool children like to relax with their Chewy Tubes at home. Three-year-old Grayson chews on a yellow Chewy Tube instead of sucking his thumb while watching a video. Four-year-old Rylee decides she wants a yellow Chewy Tube and a green Knobby Tube.*

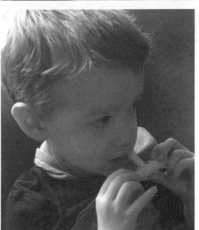

Feeding Problems and Picky Eating

Feeding problems, including picky eating, are usually very stressful for parents and their children. If your child has any of the following feeding problems, talk to your child's pediatrician:

- My child does not eat enough.

- My child wants to eat all the time.

- My child will only eat certain foods.

You may also need to work with a registered pediatric nutritionist or dietician and/or feeding therapist (such as an occupational therapist or a speech-language pathologist who specializes in feeding).

Some children do not eat what is considered enough because they have small stomachs. Remember, the size of your child's stomach is about the size of your child's fist. For these children, your child's pediatrician may recommend you feed your child small meals throughout the day. We already know this is a good practice for most of us.

Some children may not seem to eat enough because they get distracted by other things in the environment. These children may begin to feel full because they don't stay focused on the meal. Look at the environment in which your child eats. Are other people being good role models while eating? What is the conversation at the table? Are topics neutral and calm? Is calming music playing as a background, or are there other distractions such as television? Some young children *zone out* or are over stimulated by television.

Other children may not eat enough because they begin to feel sick when they eat. These may be children who have some type of food sensitivity or allergy. They may also have reflux. Infant massage can be helpful for babies with digestive problems and has been shown to improve weight gain.[267] Some children may want to eat all the time; it's important to evaluate these children for gastroesophageal reflux. I have worked with many children who have chronic reflux. When a person swallows, the esophagus is set into motion toward the stomach. This makes it impossible for the child to reflux. Therefore, a child may want to eat all the time because it stops or reduces reflux. There are also children who graze throughout the day. Some of these children have difficulty gaining weight. Grazing is not the same as eating small meals every few hours.

What To Do If My Child has Feeding Problems

Place check marks in the columns next to the problem(s) you are seeing and the things you may want to try.

PROBLEM My child:	CHECK MARK	THINGS TO TRY	CHECK MARK
Does not eat enough	☐	Provide smaller meals throughout the day; eliminate distractions from the environment; work toward a neutral, soothing environment with good role models; notice how your child is acting (for example, does he burp a lot or seem to have belly problems?); work with your child's pediatrician, registered pediatric nutritionist or dietician, and/or feeding specialist.	☐
Wants to eat all the time	☐	Have your child evaluated for possible food allergies, sensitivies, and/or reflux; work with your child's pediatrician, registered pediatric nutritionist or dietician, and/or feeding specialist.	☐

If your child is a picky eater, look for:

- Problems with airway or mouth.

- Problems with sensation in and/or around the mouth.

- Any medical issues (such as reflux or upper respiratory concerns) that may be related to the problem.

- Whether food textures were introduced on schedule.

- Behavior problems that have become related to picky eating.

What To Do if My Child is a Picky Eater

Place check marks in the columns next to the problem(s) you are seeing and the things you may want to try.

PROBLEM My child seems to have a problem with:	CHECK MARK	THINGS TO TRY	CHECK MARK
Mouth movements for eating and drinking.	☐	See a feeding specialist who knows about mouth movement (such as a speech-language pathologist or an occupational therapist who specializes in feeding).	☐
Sensation in, near, and/or around the mouth (taste, texture, temperature, smell, etc.).	☐	See a feeding specialist who knows about sensation (such as a speech-language pathologist or an occupational therapist who specializes in feeding); slowly and systematically change your child's food and liquid textures, tastes, smells, etc. over time.	☐
Gastroesophageal reflux, respiratory (airway), or other medical conditions that may be related to the problem.	☐	See your child's pediatrician and appropriate specialists. Frequently, airway problems such as a chronic stuffy nose will contribute to feeding, eating, and swallowing problems. Breathing needs to be coordinated with swallowing. Gastroesophageal reflux has been connected with chronic nasal, sinus, and ear problems, as well as asthma and voice disorders.	☐
Behavior that has become related to picky eating.	☐	See a feeding specialist who knows about behavior in addition to sensory-motor problems (such as a speech-language pathologist or an occupational therapist who specializes in feeding). Also, consider adding a behavioral specialist to your team. Applied Behavioral Analysis (ABA) specialists, psychologists, and pediatric social workers can be appropriate additions to a team when needed.	☐

If your child is a picky eater, speak with your child's pediatrician. If this is a serious concern (such as your child is not getting adequate hydration and nutrition), your child's pediatrician will usually refer you to a feeding specialist and a registered pediatric nutritionist or dietician. The feeding specialist should be someone who can evaluate the problems listed in the chart above. Therefore, you will probably see a speech-language pathologist or occupational therapist specifically trained in feeding. The registered pediatric nutritionist or dietician will guide you, the feeding specialist, and your child's pediatrician in food, liquid, and supplement selection for your child as needed.

From reading this book, you know a lot about how your child's mouth is supposed to move during feeding. If your child does not seem to have the ability to move the mouth appropriately for a feeding activity, you will need someone to evaluate this for you. A feeding specialist (such as an occupational therapist or a speech-language pathologist who specializes in feeding) can evaluate your child and provide you and your child with activities to do at home. This way your child can develop the movement needed for good feeding, eating, and drinking. In addition, you can systematically change your child's food and liquid textures to see if your child improves. For example, thickened liquids provide more information to the mouth than regular thin liquids. Your child may improve with drinking if you thicken the liquid. You can also change the texture of food by using your blender or food processor. See if your child does better if you change the texture (either thicker or thinner).

Some children also prefer to have increased or different tastes. Baby foods tend to be very bland. Many baby formulas have a medicine-like taste. Babies typically prefer sweet and salty tastes, but you don't want to add too much sugar or salt to the food. However, you can present foods that tend to be on sweet or salty side naturally (such as carrots, squash, fruit, and fish when your child is ready). See Food and Liquid Introduction Checklist: Birth to 24 Months in Chapter 1. As your child gets older, you can add tastes you have in your diet (such as garlic, onion, cinnamon, and other appropriate spices), particularly if your child likes increased taste. If you are breastfeeding, your baby is likely getting many different tastes already. You can add breast milk to cereal to see if your baby (around 6 months) prefers that combination over baby cereal made with water only.

It's also important to see if your child has any medical problems that may cause him to be picky. A child who has reflux may realize at some level certain foods make him feel sick. However, he may not know which foods are causing the problem. This can also change from day to day. Reflux and other digestive problems may provide at least part of the explanation for picky eating in some children. Additionally, gastroesophageal reflux has been connected with chronic nasal, sinus, and ear problems, as well as asthma and voice disorders.

Frequently, airway problems such as a chronic stuffy nose will contribute to feeding, eating, and swallowing problems. Breathing needs to be coordinated with swallowing. If your child has nasal or sinus problems, this can change the taste of foods. Have you noticed that food tastes different when you have a sinus infection or cold? Therefore, it's very important to take care of any nasal or sinus problems your child may be having. The smell of food is an important aspect of being able to experience taste. We basically taste sweet, salty, sour, savory, and bitter with the tongue. It's the smell and intensity of food that seems to allow us to taste the difference between flavors such as cherry and strawberry. When children are picky eaters, it can often be the smell of the food that does not appeal to them. If they can't tolerate the smell of a food, they won't want it in their mouths. So, in therapy, I usually begin by looking at whether the child likes the smell of the food or not before moving to the mouth to taste the food.

If your child is having difficulties accepting particular food or liquid smells, tastes, textures, etc., a food record is an important starting point. You need a record of at least 3 full days of everything your child eats and drinks. Once you have this, you can begin to systematically make some small changes in your child's diet with the help of a feeding specialist (such as an occupational therapist or a speech-language pathologist who specializes in feeding) and registered pediatric dietician or nutritionist.

Food and Liquid Record

Record the food and fluid, with approximate amounts, consumed by your child below. Enter the date next to the appropriate day.

	BREAKFAST	LUNCH	DINNER	SNACKS
DAY 1:				
DAY 2:				
DAY 3:				

My Child's Eating and Drinking Patterns

Look at your child's food and liquid record, and take note of any patterns. Use the chart below to help you discover his or her individual preferences. You may also realize during this process that your child is doing better than you thought. Work with a feeding therapist (such as an occupational therapist or a speech-language pathologist who specializes in feeding), registered pediatric dietician or nutritionist, and your child's pediatrician as needed.

FOOD AND LIQUID CHARACTERISTICS	WHAT IS SIMILAR ABOUT MY CHILD'S FOODS AND LIQUIDS?	WHAT COULD WE TRY?
Taste		
Smell		
Texture		
Temperature		
Color		
Shape		
Other		

In addition to mouth movement, sensation, airway, and medical problems, behavioral issues quickly become associated with feeding problems. This occurs because behavior is a way of communicating. If your child cannot let you know something in words, he will let you know through behavior and body language. In addition to a feeding specialist and registered pediatric dietician or nutritionist, consider adding a behavioral specialist to your team if needed. Applied Behavioral Analysis (ABA) specialists, psychologists, and pediatric social workers can be appropriate additions to a feeding team.

I am often concerned when parents and professionals assume picky eating is purely a behavioral problem. It's important to look at what your child's behavior is communicating. This way, you can find ways to change the situation and let your child know you understand his or her communication. Also, involve your child in the food preparation process. This may seem a bit odd for you to do with a very young child, but he is learning a lot from what is happening in the environment around him. It helps the child to become part of the process.

It can be as simple as having your child sit in the feeding chair as you prepare some of the meal. Your child does not need to sit there the entire time. You can show your child the foods you are about to prepare and talk about the food. Let him see, smell, and touch the food. Praise him for doing this. Give your child a choice of which food you are going to prepare. Even very small babies (6-month-old children) make choices with their eyes and body language. For example, you can say, "Kyle, pick one for Mommy or Daddy to cook," as you show him broccoli and asparagus. You let him look at, smell, and touch the one he picks. Praise him for helping you.

Many children like to go to the grocery store with Mom and Dad. This is a great time to talk about the foods you are picking out for your family meals. Your child can help you make some choices. Of course, you will be offering healthy food choices that support your family's nutritional needs. For example, you could say, "Erica, should we get apples or pears?"

Some parents also give their children too many choices of foods. When giving choices, limit your choices to 2 items at first. Too many choices can overwhelm your child. I once worked with a mom who had 15 jars of baby food on the table as choices for her baby. This was very overwhelming for the child and for Mom. Having your child make food choices and becoming involved in food preparation is a way to gain cooperation and participation. This can help your child develop a wonderful relationship with food for life. As you feed your child, remember meals are social experiences. Take your time. Talk to your child. Have some food to eat or liquid to drink with your child. This will help you and your child pace the meal, another important life skill.

Parents also need to remember their child may not like a food the first time he or she tastes it. Do you like every food the first time you taste it? How many times does it take? You may need to provide your child with 10 to 15 exposures of a food to help him accommodate to the smell, taste, and/or texture of a food. Be patient with this process, and do not force-feed your child. If your child initially spits out a food, don't assume he will never like it. This may only be his reaction to something new. Also, if you react by getting upset with your child when he spits out food, this can inadvertently reinforce the spitting.

There are a number of books written for parents addressing picky eating and nutrition. Here are a few:

- *Adventures in Veggieland: Help Your Kids Learn to Love Vegetables with 100 Easy Activities and Recipes* by Melanie Potock [268]

- *Baby Self-Feeding: Solid Food Solutions to Create Lifelong, Healthy Eating Habits* by Nancy Ripton and Melanie Potock [269]

- *Child of Mine: Feeding with Love and Good Sense* by Ellyn Satter [270]

- *Happy Mealtimes with Happy Kids: How to Teach Your Child about the Joy of Food* by Melanie Potock [271]

- *Helping Your Child with Extreme Picky Eating: A Step-by-Step Guide for Overcoming Selective Eating, Food Aversion, and Feeding Disorders* by Katja Rowell and Jenny McGlothlin [272]

- *How to Get Your Kid to Eat … But Not Too Much* by Ellen Satter [273]

- *Just Take a Bite: Easy, Effective, Answers to Food Aversion and Eating Challenges* by Lori Ernsperger, and Tania Stegen-Hanson [274]

- *Raising a Healthy, Happy Eater: A Stage-by-Stage Guide to Setting Your Child on the Path to Adventurous Eating* by Nimali Fernando and Melanie Potock [275]

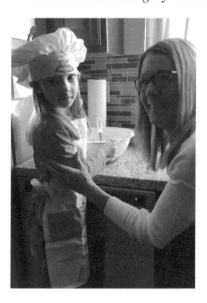 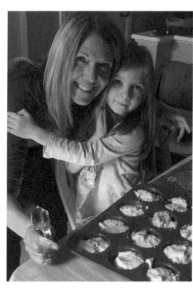

Photo 4.18: *Chef Rylee (age 5) makes muffins with her grandmother Diane.*

References

1. Karp, H. (2002). *The Happiest Baby on the Block*. New York, NY: Bantam Dell, 4.

2. Morris, S.E. (2003). *A Longitudinal Study of Feeding and Pre-Speech Skills from Birth to Three Years* (unpublished research study). VA: New Visions.

3. Morris, S.E., & Klein, M.D. (2000). *Pre-Feeding Skills: A Comprehensive Resource for Mealtime Development* (2nd ed.). Austin, TX: Pro Ed, 51-53, 71, 525-529, 697-711.

4. Morris, S.E., & Klein, M.D. (1987). *Pre-Feeding skills: A Comprehensive Resource for Feeding Development*. Tucson, AZ: Therapy Skill Builders, 305-306.

5. Morris, S.E. (1985). "Developmental Implications for the Management of Feeding Problems in Neurologically Impaired Infants. *Semin Speech Lang, 6*(4): 293-315.

6. Bahr, D., & Gatto, K. (2017, Nov.). *Mouth and Airway Development, Disorders, Assessment, and Treatment: Birth to Age 7*. Los Angeles, CA: American Speech-Language-Hearing Convention.

7. Bahr, D. (2010). *Nobody Ever Told Me (or My Mother) That! Everything from Bottles and Breathing to Healthy Speech Development*. Arlington, TX: Sensory World.

8. Bahr, D.C. (2001). *Oral Motor Assessment and Treatment: Ages and Stages*. Boston, MA: Allyn and Bacon, 5, 17-20, 44-45, 121-133, 147.

9. Lau, C. (2015). "Development of Suck and Swallow Mechanisms in Infants." *Ann Nutr Metab, 66*(suppl. 5): 7–14.

10. Oetter, P., Richter, E.W., & Frick, S.M. (1995). *M.O.R.E.: Integrating the Mouth with Sensory and Postural Functions* (2nd ed.). Hugo, MN: PDP Press, Inc., 8, 20, 27.

11. Winstock, A. (2005). *Eating & Drinking Difficulties in Children: A Guide for Practitioners*. Oxon, UK: Speechmark Publishing, Ltd.

12. Montagu, A. (1986). *Touching: The Human Significance of the Skin* (3rd ed.). New York: Harper & Row, Publishers, 84.

13. American Dental Association (2012). *Primary Tooth Development*. Retrieved from http://www.mouthhealthy.org/en/az-topics/e/eruption-charts.

14. Kent, R.D. (1999). "Motor Control: Neurophysiology and Functional Development." In A.J. Caruso and E.A. Strand (Eds.), *Clinical Management of Motor Speech Disorders in Children* (pp. 29-71). New York: Thieme Medical Publishers.

15. Eisenberg, A., Murkoff, H.E., & Hathaway, S.E. (1989). *What to Expect the First Year.* New York: Workman Publishing.

16. Eisenberg, A., Murkoff, H.E., & Hathaway, S.E. (1994). *What to Expect: The Toddler Years.* New York: Workman Publishing.

17. Uddin, L.Q., Iacoboni, M., Lange, C., & Keenan, J.P. (2007). "The Self and Social Cognition: The Role of Cortical Midline Structures and Mirror Neurons." *Trends Cogn Sci, 11*(4): 153-157.

18. Miall, R.C. (2003). "Connecting Mirror Neurons and Forward Models." *Neuroreport, 14*(17): 2135-2137.

19. Heyes, C. (2010). "Where do Mirror Neurons Come From?" *Neuro Biobehav Rev, 34*(4): 575-583.

20. Morris, S.E. (2003). *A Longitudinal Study of Feeding and Pre-Speech Skills from Birth to Three Years* (unpublished research study). VA: New Visions.

21. Morris, S.E., & Klein, M.D. (2000). *Pre-Feeding skills: A Comprehensive Resource for Mealtime Development* (2nd ed.). Austin, TX: Pro Ed.

22. Widström, A.M., Lilja, G., Aaltomaa-Michalias, P., Dahllöf, A., Lintula, M., & Nissen, E. (2011). "Newborn Behaviour to Locate the Breast when Skin-to-Skin: A Possible Method for Enabling Early Self-Regulation." *Acta paediatrica, 100*(1): 79-85.

23. Girish, M., Mujawar, N., Gotmare, P., Paul, N., Punia, S., & Pandey, P. (2013). "Impact and Feasibility of Breast Crawl in a Tertiary Care Hospital." *J Perinatol, 33*(4): 288-291.

24. Heidarzadeh, M., Hakimi, S., Habibelahi, A., Mohammadi, M., & Shahrak, S.P. (2016). "Comparison of Breast Crawl Between Infants Delivered by Vaginal Delivery and Cesarean Section." *Breastfeed Med, 11*(6): 305-308.

25. McDonald, S.J., & Middleton, P. (2008). "Effect of Timing of Umbilical Cord Clamping of Term Infants on Maternal and Neonatal Outcomes." *Cochrane Database Syst Rev, 2*(2).

26. Guilleminault, C., & Huang, Y.S. (2017). "From Oral Facial Dysfunction to Dysmorphism and the Onset of Pediatric OSA." *Sleep Medicine Reviews.*

27. Abreu, R.R., Rocha, R.L., Lamounier, J.A., & Guerra, Â.F.M. (2008b). "Etiology, Clinical Manifestations and Concurrent Findings in Mouth-Breathing Children." *Jornal de Pediatria, 84*(6): 529-535.

28. Guilleminault, C., & Sullivan, S.S. (2014). "Towards Restoration of Continuous Nasal Breathing as the Ultimate Treatment Goal in Pediatric Obstructive Sleep Apnea." *Enliven, 1*(1): 1-5.

29. Lee, S.H., Choi, J.H., Shin, C., Lee, H.M., Kwon, S.Y., & Lee, S.H. (2007). "How Does Open-Mouth Breathing Influence Upper Airway Anatomy?" *Laryngoscope, 117*, 1102–1106.

30. Lee, S., Guilleminault, C., Chiu, H., & Sullivan, S.S. (2015). "Mouth Breathing, 'Nasal Disuse,' and Pediatric Sleep-Disordered Breathing." *Sleep Breath, 19*(4): 1257-1264.

31. Trevarthen, C. (1979). "Communication and Cooperation in Early Infancy: A Description of Primary Intersubjectivity." In M. Bullowa (Ed.) *Before Speech* (pp. 321-347). New York, NY: Cambridge University Press.

32. Morris, S.E., & Klein, M.D. (2000). *Pre-Feeding Skills: A Comprehensive Resource for Mealtime Development* (2nd ed.). Austin, TX: Pro Ed, 69.

33. Feig, C. (2011). *Exclusive Breastfeeding for Six Months Best for Babies Everywhere.* Geneva, Switzerland: World Health Organization. Retrieved from http://www.who.int/mediacentre/news/statements/2011/breastfeeding_20110115/en/.

34. Kramer M.S., & Kakuma R. (2012). "Optimal Duration of Exclusive Breastfeeding." *Cochrane Database Syst Rev, 8* (CD003517).

35. Stevenson, R.D., & Allaire, J.H. (1991). "The Development of Normal Feeding and Swallowing." *Pediatric Clinics of North America, 38*(6): 1439-1453.

36. Tinanoff, N., & Palmer, C.A. (2000). "Dietary Determinants of Dental Caries and Dietary Recommendations for Preschool Children." *Journal Public Health Dent, 60*(3): 197-206.

37. Potock, M. (n.d.). "Why You May Want to Skip the Sippy Cup for Your Baby." *Parents.* Retrieved from https://www.parents.com/baby/feeding/center/why-you-may-want-to-skip-the-sippy-cup-for-your-baby/.

38. Potock, M. (2014, Jan). "Step Away from the Sippy Cup!" *The ASHA Leader Blog.* Retrieved from https://blog.asha.org/2014/01/09/step-away-from-the-sippy-cup/.

39. Potock, M. (2017, Feb). "Sippy Cups: 3 Reasons to Skip Them and What to Offer Instead." *The ASHA Leader Blog.* Retrieved from https://blog.asha.org/2017/02/28/sippy-cups-3-reasons-to-skip-them-and-what-to-offer-instead/.

40. Tinanoff, N., & Palmer, C.A. (2000). "Dietary Determinants of Dental Caries and Dietary Recommendations for Preschool Children." *Journal Public Health Dent, 60*(3): 197-206.

41. Potock, M. (n.d.). "Why You May Want to Skip the Sippy Cup for your Baby." *Parents.* Retrieved from https://www.parents.com/baby/feeding/center/why-you-may-want-to-skip-the-sippy-cup-for-your-baby/.

42. Potock, M. (2014, Jan). "Step Away from the Sippy Cup!" *The ASHA Leader Blog.* Retrieved from https://blog.asha.org/2014/01/09/step-away-from-the-sippy-cup/.

43. Potock, M. (2017, Feb). "Sippy Cups: 3 Reasons to Skip Them and What to Offer Instead." *The ASHA Leader Blog.* Retrieved from https://blog.asha.org/2017/02/28/sippy-cups-3-reasons-to-skip-them-and-what-to-offer-instead/.

44. Satter, E. (2000). *Child of Mine: Feeding with Love and Good Sense, Revised.* Boulder, CO: Bull Publishing Company, 250-251.

45. Stoppard, M. (1998). *First Foods.* New York: DK Publishing, Inc., 14-15.

46. Morris, S.E., & Klein, M.D. (2000). *Pre-Feeding Skills: A Comprehensive Resource for Mealtime Development* (2nd ed.). Austin, TX: Pro Ed, 697-711.

47. Samuels, M. & Samuels, N. (1991). *The Well Baby Book: A Comprehensive Manual of Baby Care, from Conception to Age Four.* New York: Summit Books, 162.

48. Huggins, K. (1999). *The Nursing Mother's Companion* (4th ed.). Boston: The Harvard Common Press, 31.

49. Cameron, S.L., Taylor, R.W., & Heath, A.L.M. (2015). "Development and Pilot Testing of Baby-Led Introduction to Solids - A Version of Baby-Led Weaning Modified to Address Concerns about Iron Deficiency, Growth Faltering, and Choking." *BMC Pediatr, 15*(1): 99.

50. Arden, M.A., & Abbott, R.L. (2015). "Experiences of Baby-Led Weaning: Trust, Control and Renegotiation." *Matern Child Nut, 11*(4): 829-844.

51. Cameron, S.L., Heath, A.L.M., & Taylor, R.W. (2012). "How Feasible is Baby-Led Weaning as an Approach to Infant Feeding? A Review of the Evidence." *Nutrients, 4*(11): 1575-1609.

52. Brown, A., & Lee, M. (2013). "An Exploration of Experiences of Mothers Following a Baby-Led Weaning Style: Developmental Readiness for Complementary Foods." *Matern Child Nut, 9*(2): 233-243.

53. Potock, M. (2018). *Adventures in Veggieland: Help Your Kids Learn to Love Vegetables with 100 Easy Activities and Recipes.* New York: The Experiment, LLC.

54. Overland, L.L., & Merkel-Walsh, R. (2015). *A Sensory Motor Approach to Feeding.* Charleston, SC: TalkTools.

55. Ripton, N., & Potock, M. (2016). *Baby Self-Feeding: Solid Food Solutions to Create Lifelong, Healthy Eating Habits.* Beverly, MA: Fairwinds Press.

56. Rapley, G., & Murkett, T. (2010). *Baby-Led Weaning: The Essential Guide to Introducing Solid Foods and Helping Your Baby Grow Up a Happy and Confident Eater.* New York: The Experiment, LLC.

57. Satter, E. (2000). *Child of Mine: Feeding with Love and Good Sense, Revised.* Boulder, CO: Bull Publishing Company.

58. Potock, M. (2010). *Happy Mealtimes with Happy Kids: How to Teach your Child About the Joy of Food.* Longmont, CO: My Munch Bug Publishing.

59. Rowell, K., & McGlothlin, J. (2015). *Helping Your Child with Extreme Picky Eating: A Step-by-Step Guide for Overcoming Selective Eating, Food Aversion, and Feeding Disorders.* Oakland, CA: New Harbinger Publications, Inc.

60. Satter, E. (1987). *How to Get Your Kid to Eat ... But Not Too Much.* Boulder, CO: Bull Publishing Company.

61. Ernsperger, L., & Stegen-Hanson, T. (2004). *Just Take a Bite: Easy, Effective, Answers to Food Aversion and Eating Challenges!* Arlington, TX: Future Horizons Inc.

62. Bahr, D. (2010). *Nobody Ever Told Me (or My Mother) That! Everything from Bottles and Breathing to Healthy Speech Development.* Arlington, TX: Sensory World.

63. Morris, S.E., & Klein, M.D. (2000). *Pre-Feeding Skills: A Comprehensive Resource for Mealtime Development* (2nd ed.). Austin, TX: Pro Ed.

64. Bly, L. (1994). *Motor Skills Acquisition in the First Year: An Illustrated Guide to Normal Development.* San Antonio, TX: Therapy Skill Builders. 1-153.

65. Dargassies, S.S.A. (1977). *Neurological Development in the Full-Term and Premature Neonate.* Excerpta Medica.

66. Vulpe, S.G. (1994). *Vulpe Assessment Battery – Revised: Developmental Assessment, Performance Analysis, Individualized Programming for the Atypical Child.* New York: Slosson Educational Publications.

67. Johnson-Martin, N.M., Attermeier, S.M., & Hacker, B.J. (2004). *The Carolina Curriculum for Infants & Toddlers with Special Needs* (3rd ed.). Baltimore, MD: Paul H. Brookes Publishing Company.

68. Mitchell, E.A., & Krous, H.F. (2015). "Sudden Unexpected Death in Infancy: A Historical Perspective." *Journal of Paediatric Child Health, 51*(1): 108-112.

69. Task Force on Sudden Infant Death Syndrome. (2011). "SIDS and Other Sleep-Related Infant Deaths: Expansion of Recommendations for a Safe Infant Sleeping Environment." *Pediatrics, 128*(5): e1341-1367.

70. Fleming, P.J., Blair, P.S., & Pease, A. (2015). "Sudden Unexpected Death in Infancy: Aetiology, Pathophysiology, Epidemiology and Prevention in 2015." *Arc Dis Child*, 100(10): 984-988.

71. Mitchell, E.A., & Blair, P.S. (2012). "SIDS Prevention: 3000 Lives Saved but We Can Do Better." *NZ Med J (Online)*, 125(1359): 50.

72. Grillon, C., Pine, D.S., Baas, J.M., Lawley, M., Ellis, V., & Charney, D.S. (2006). "Cortisol and DHEA-S are Associated with Startle Potentiation During Aversive Conditioning in Humans." *Psychopharmacology, 186*(3): 434-441.

73. Brain Sync (n.d.). *Moro Reflex*. Retrieved from http://www.brain-sync.net/reflexes-2/moro/.

74. Move, Play, Thrive (n.d.). *Moro Reflex*. Retrieved from https://www.moveplaythrive.com/articles-by-move-play-thrive/unintegrated-reflexes/37-moro-reflex.

75. Bonuck, K.A., Chervin, R.D, Cole, T.J., Emond, A., Henderson, J., Xu, L., & Freeman, K. (2011). "Prevalence and Persistence of Sleep Disordered Breathing Symptoms in Young Children: A 6-Year Population-Based Cohort Study." *SLEEP, 34*(7): 875-884.

76. Bonuck, K., Freeman, K., Chervin, R.D., & Xu, L. (2012). "Sleep-Disordered Breathing in a Population-Based Cohort: Behavioral Outcomes at 4 and 7 Years." *Pediatrics, 129*(4): 1-9.

77. Guilleminault, C., & Akhtar, F. (2015). "Pediatric Sleep-Disordered Breathing: New Evidence on Its Development." *Sleep Med Rev, 24*, 46-56.

78. Guilleminault, C., & Huang, Y.S. (2017). "From Oral Facial Dysfunction to Dysmorphism and the Onset of Pediatric OSA." *Sleep Medicine Reviews*.

79. Guilleminault, C., Huang, Y.S., Monteyrol, P.J., Sato, R., Quo, S., & Lin, C.H. (2013). "Critical Role of Myofascial Reeducation in Pediatric Sleep-Disordered Breathing." *Sleep Med, 14*(6): 518-525.

80. Bly, L. (1994). *Motor Skills Acquisition in the First Year: An Illustrated Guide to Normal Development*. San Antonio, TX: Therapy Skill Builders. 1-153.

81. Vulpe, S.G. (1994). *Vulpe Assessment Battery – Revised: Developmental Assessment, Performance Analysis, Individualized Programming for the Atypical Child*. New York: Slosson Educational Publications.

82. Bahr, D.C. (2001). *Oral Motor Assessment and Treatment: Ages and Stages*. (Boston: Allyn and Bacon), 4-7.

83. Bahr, D. (2010). *Nobody Ever Told Me (or My Mother) That! Everything from Bottles and Breathing to Healthy Speech Development*. Arlington, TX: Sensory World.

84. Love, R.J., & Webb, W.G. (1996). *Neurology for the Speech-Language Pathologist*. (3rd ed.) Boston: Butterworth-Heinemann, 287-293.

85. Morris, S.E., & Klein, M.D. (1987). *Pre-Feeding Skills: A Comprehensive Resource for Feeding Development*. Tucson: Therapy Skill Builders, 26-27.

86. Morris, S.E., & Klein. M.D. (2000). *Pre-Feeding Skills: A Comprehensive Resource for Mealtime Development* (2nd ed.). Austin, TX: Pro Ed, 71, 697-711.

87. Samuels, M., & Samuels, N. (1991). *The Well Baby Book: A Comprehensive Manual of Baby Care, from Conception to Age Four*. New York: Summit Books, 142.

88. Tuchman, D.N., & Walter, R.S.(1994). *Disorders of Feeding and Swallowing in Infants and Children: Pathophysiology, Diagnosis, and Treatment*. San Diego: Singular Publishing Group, 29-31.

89. Montagu, A. (1986). *Touching: The Human Significance of the Skin* (3rd ed.). New York: Harper & Row, Publishers, 69-95.

90. Stevenson, R.D., & Allaire, J.H. (1991). *The Development of Normal Feeding and Swallowing*. Pediatric Clinics of North America, 38(6): 1439-1453.

91. Montagu, A. (1986). *Touching: The Human Significance of the Skin* (3rd ed.). New York: Harper & Row, Publishers, 82.

92. Oetter, P., Richter, E.W., & Frick, S.M. (1995) *M.O.R.E.: Integrating the Mouth with Sensory and Postural Functions* (2nd ed.). Hugo, MN: PDP Press, Inc., 21.

93. Morris, S.E., & Klein, M.D. (2000). *Pre-Feeding Skills: A Comprehensive Resource for Mealtime Development* (2nd ed.) Austin, TX: Pro Ed, 69.

94. Bahr, D.C. (2001). *Oral Motor Assessment and Treatment: Ages and Stages*. Boston: Allyn and Bacon, 4-7.

95. Bahr, D. (2010). *Nobody Ever Told Me (or My Mother) That! Everything from Bottles and Breathing to Healthy Speech Development*. Arlington, TX: Sensory World.

96. Morris, S.E., & Klein, M.D. (1987). *Pre-Feeding Skills: A Comprehensive Resource for Feeding Development*. Tucson, AZ: Therapy Skill Builders, 26-27.

97. Tuchman, D.N., & Walter, R.S. (1994). *Disorders of Feeding and Swallowing in Infants and Children: Pathophysiology, Diagnosis, and Treatment*. San Diego: Singular Publishing Group, 29-31.

98. Genna, C.W., & Sandora, L. (2017). "Breastfeeding: Normal Sucking and Swallowing." In C.W. Genna (Ed.), *Supporting Sucking Skills in Breastfeeding Infants* (3rd ed., pp. 1-48). Woodhaven, NY: Jones and Bartlett Learning.

99. Elad, D., Kozlovsky, P., Blum, O., Laine, A.F., Ming, J.P. Botzer, E., Dollberg, S., Zelicovich, M., & Sira L.B. (2014, Apr.). "Biomechanics of Milk Extraction During Breast-Feeding." *Proceedings of the National Academy of Sciences for the United Stated of America, 111*(14). 5230-5235.

100. Geddes, D.T., Kent, J.C., Mitoulas, L.R., & Hartmann, P.E. (2008). "Tongue Movement and Intra-Oral Vacuum in Breastfeeding Infants." *Early Hum Dev, 84*(7): 471-477.

101. Gomes, C.F., Trezza, E., Murade, E., & Padovani, C.R. (2006). "Surface Electromyography of Facial Muscles During Natural and Artificial Feeding of Infants." *Jornal de Pediatria, 82*(2): 103-109.

102. Inoue, N., Sakashita, R., & Kamegai, T. (1995). "Reduction of Masseter Muscle Activity in Bottle-Fed Babies." *Early Hum Dev, 42*(3): 185-193.

103. Moral, A., Bolibar, I., Seguranyes, G., Ustrell, J, Sebastia, G., Martínez-Barba, C., & Ríos, J. (2010). "Mechanics of Sucking: Comparison Between Bottle Feeding and Breastfeeding." *BMC Pediatrics, 10*(6): 1- 8.

104. Miller, J.L., & Kang, S.M. (2007). "Preliminary Ultrasound Observation of Lingual Movement Patterns During Nutritive Versus Non-Nutritive Sucking in a Premature Infant." *Dysphagia, 22*(2): 150-160.

105. Nyqvist, K.H., Färnstrand, C., Eeg-Olofsson, K.E., & Ewald, U. (2001). "Early Oral Behaviour in Preterm Infants During Breastfeeding: An Electromyographic Study." *Acta Paediatr, 90*(6): 658-663.

106. Oetter, P., Richter, E.W., & Frick S.M. (1995). *M.O.R.E.: Integrating the Mouth with Sensory and Postural Functions* (2nd ed.). Hugo, MN: PDP Press, Inc.

107. Montagu, A. (1986). *Touching: The Human Significance of the Skin* (3rd ed.). New York: Harper and Row Publishers, 85.

108. Moral, A., Bolibar, I., Seguranyes, G., Ustrell, J, Sebastia, G., Martínez-Barba, C., & Ríos, J. (2010). "Mechanics of Sucking: Comparison Between Bottle Feeding and Breastfeeding." *BMC Pediatrics, 10*(6): 1- 8.

109. Silveira, L.M.D., Prade, L.S., Ruedell, A.M., Haeffner, L.S.B., & Weinmann, A.R.M. (2013). "Influence of Breastfeeding on Children's Oral Skills." *Revista de Saúde Pública, 47*(1): 37-43.

110. Bartick, M., & Reinhold, A. (2010). "The Burden of Suboptimal Breastfeeding in the United States: A Pediatric Cost Analysis." *Pediatrics, 125*(5): e1048-e1056.

111. Montagu, A. (1986). *Touching: The Human Significance of the Skin* (3rd ed.). New York: Harper and Row Publishers, 83.

112. Bueno, S.B., Bittar, T.O., Vazquez, F.D.L., Meneghim, M.C., & Pereira, A.C. (2013). "Association of Breastfeeding, Pacifier Use, Breathing Pattern and Malocclusions in Preschoolers." *Dental Press J Orthod, 18*(1): 30e1-30e6.

113. Warren, J.J., Levy, S.M., Kirchner, H.L., Nowak, A.J., & Bergus, G.R. (2001). "Pacifier Use and the Occurrence of Otitis Media in the First Year of Life." *Pediatr Dent, 23*(2): 103-108.

114. Cheng, M.C., Enlow, D.H., Papsidero, M., Broadbent, B.H. Jr, Oyen, O., & Sabat, M. (1988). "Developmental Effects of Impaired Breathing in the Face of the Growing Child." *Angle Orthod, 58*, 309– 320.

115. Guilleminault, C., & Huang, Y.S. (2017). "From Oral Facial Dysfunction to Dysmorphism and the Onset of Pediatric OSA." *Sleep Med Rev.*

116. Lundberg, J.O.N., & Weitzberg, E. (1999). "Nasal Nitric Oxide in Man." *Thorax, 54*(10): 947-952.

117. Marangu, D., Jowi, C., Aswani, J., Wambani, S., & Nduati, R. (2014). "Prevalence and Associated Factors of Pulmonary Hypertension in Kenyan Children with Adenoid or Adenotonsillar Hypertrophy." *Int J Pediatr Otorhinolaryngol, 78*(8): 1381-1386.

118. Schlenker, W.L., Jennings, B.D., Jeiroudi, M.T., & Caruso, J.M. (2000). "The Effects of Chronic Absence of Active Nasal Respiration on the Growth of the Skull: A Pilot Study." *Am J Orthod Dentofacial Orthop, 117*(6): 706-713.

119. Page, D.C., Sr. (2003). "'Real' Early Orthodontic Treatment: From Birth to Age 8." *Funct Orthod: J Funct Jaw Orthop, 20*(1-2): 48-58.

120. Aniansson, G., Alm, B., Andersson, B., Håkansson, A., Larsson, P., Nylén, O., Peterson, H., Rignér, P., Svanborg, M., Sabharwal, H., et al. (1994). "A Prospective Cohort Study on Breast-Feeding and Otitis Media in Swedish Infants." *Pediatr Infect Dis J, 13*(3): 183-188.

121. Watkins, C.J., Leeder, S.R., & Corkhill, R.T. (1979). "The Relationship Between Breast and Bottle Feeding and Respiratory Illness in the First Year of Life." *J Epidemiol Community Health, 33*(3): 180-182.

122. Gerstein H.C. (1994). "Cow's Milk Exposure and Type I Diabetes Mellitus. A Critical Overview of the Clinical Literature." *Diabetes Care, 17*(1): 13-9.

123. Barlow, B., Santulli, T.V., Heird, W.C., Pitt, J., Blanc, W.A., & Schullinger, J.N. (1974). "An Experimental Study of Acute Neonatal Enterocolitis - The Importance of Breast Milk." *J Pediatr Surg, 9*(5): 587-595.

124. Saarinen U.M., & Kajosaari M. (1995). "Breastfeeding as Prophylaxis Against Atopic Disease: Prospective Follow-Up Study Until 17 Years Old." *Lancet, 346*(8982): 1065-1069.

125. Cullinan, T.R., & Saunder D.I. (1983). "Prediction of Infant Hospital Admission Risk." *Arch Dis Child, 68*, 423-427.

126. Mitchell, E.A., Scragg, R., Stewart, A.W., Becroft, D.M., Taylor, B.J., Ford, R.P., ... & Roberts, A.P. (1991). "Results from the First Year of the New Zealand Cot Death Study." *NZ Med J, 104*(906): 71-76.

127. Pottenger, F.M., & Krohn, B. (1950). "Influence of Breast Feeding on Facial Development." *Arch Pediatr, 67*(10): 454-461.

128. Robinson, S., & Naylor, S.R. (1963). "The Effects of Late Weaning on the Deciduous Incisor Teeth: A Pilot Survey." *Brit Dent. J, 115*, 250-252.

129. Nizel, A.E. (1975). "Nursing Bottle Syndrome: Rampant Dental Caries in Young Children." *Nutr News*, 38, 1-7.

130. Broad, F.E. (1972). "The Effects of Infant Feeding on Speech Quality." NZ Med J, 76, 28-31.

131. Broad, F.E. (1975). "Further Studies on the Effects of Infant Feeding on Speech Quality." *NZ Med J, 82*, 373- 376.

132. Bertrand, F.R. (1968). "The Relationship of Prolonged Breast Feeding to Facial Features." *Cent Afr J Med, (14)*: 226-227.

133. Santos-Neto, E.T., Oliveira, A.E., Barbosa, R.W., Zandonade, E., & Oliveira, L. (2012). "The Influence of Sucking Habits on Occlusion Development in the First 36 Months." *Dental Press J Orthod, 17*(4): 96-104.

134. Peres, K.G., Cascaes, A.M., Nascimento, G.G., & Victora, C.G. (2015). "Effect of Breastfeeding on Malocclusions: A Systematic Review and Meta-Analysis." *Acta Paediatr, 104*(S467): 54-61.

135. Peres, K.G., Cascaes, A.M., Peres, M.A., Demarco, F.F., Santos, I.S., Matijasevich, A., & Barros, A.J. (2015). "Exclusive Breastfeeding and Risk of Dental Malocclusion." *Pediatrics, 136*(1): e60-e67.

136. Sabuncuoglu, O. (2013). "Understanding the Relationships Between Breastfeeding, Malocclusion, ADHD, Sleep-Disordered Breathing and Traumatic Dental Injuries." *Medical Hypotheses, 80*(3): 315-320.

137. Bueno, S.B., Bittar, T.O., Vazquez, F.D.L., Meneghim, M.C., & Pereira, A.C. (2013). "Association of Breastfeeding, Pacifier Use, Breathing Pattern and Malocclusions in Preschoolers." *Dental Press J Orthod, 18*(1): 30e1-30e6.

138. Page, D.C., Sr. (2003). "'Real' Early Orthodontic Treatment: From Birth to Age 8." *Funct Orthod: J Funct Jaw Orthop, 20*(1-2): 48-58.

139. Page, D.C., Sr. (2003). "'Real' Early Orthodontic Treatment: From Birth to Age 8." *Funct Orthod: J Funct Jaw Orthop, 20*(1-2): 54.

140. Paunio, P., Rautava, P., & Sillanpää, M. (1993). "The Finnish Family Competence Study: The Effects of Living Conditions on Sucking Habits in 3-Year-Old Finnish Children and the Association Between These Habits and Dental Occlusion." *Acta Odontol Scand 51*(1): 23-29.

141. Davis, D.W., & Bell, P.A. (1991). "Infant Feeding Practices and Occlusal Outcomes: A Longitudinal Study." *J Can Dent Assoc, 57*(7): 593-594.

142. Paunio, P., Rautava, P., & Sillanpaa, M. (1993). "The Finnish Family Competence Study: The Effects of Living Conditions on Sucking Habits in 3-Year-Old Finnish Children and the Association Between These Habits and Dental Occlusion." *Acta Odontol Scand, 51*(1): 23-29.

143. Peres, K.G., Cascaes, A.M., Nascimento, G.G., & Victora, C.G. (2015). "Effect of Breastfeeding on Malocclusions: A Systematic Review and Meta-Analysis." *Acta Paediatr, 104*(S467): 54-61.

144. Peres, K.G., Cascaes, A.M., Peres, M.A., Demarco, F.F., Santos, I.S., Matijasevich, A., & Barros, A.J. (2015). "Exclusive Breastfeeding and Risk of Dental Malocclusion." *Pediatrics, 136*(1): e60-e67.

145. Sabuncuoglu, O. (2013). "Understanding the Relationships Between Breastfeeding, Malocclusion, ADHD, Sleep-Disordered Breathing and Traumatic Dental Injuries." *Medical Hypotheses, 80*(3): 315-320.

146. Bueno, S.B., Bittar, T.O., Vazquez, F.D.L., Meneghim, M.C., & Pereira, A.C. (2013). "Association of Breastfeeding, Pacifier Use, Breathing Pattern and Malocclusions in Preschoolers." *Dental Press J Orthod, 18*(1): 30e1-30e6.

147. Ogarrd, B., Larsson, E., & Lindsten, R. (1994). "The Effect of Sucking Habits, Cohort, Sex, Inter-Canine Arch Widths, and Breast or Bottle Feeding on Posterior Crossbite in Norwegian and Swedish 3-Year-Old Children." *Am J Orthod Dentofacial Orthop, 106*(2): 161-166.

148. Montagu, A. (1986). Touching: *The Human Significance of the Skin* (3rd ed.). New York: Harper and Row Publishers, 69-95.

149. Kimball, E.R. (1968, June). "How I Get Mothers to Breastfeed." *Physician's Management* (OB/GYN'S Supplement).

150. Hoefer, C., & Hardy, M.C. (1929). "Later Development of Breast Fed and Artificially Fed Infants." *JAMA, 96,* 615-619.

151. Horwood, I.J., & Ferguson, D.M. (1998). "Breastfeeding and Later Cognitive and Academic Outcomes." *Pediatrics, 101*(1): E9.

152. Hoefer, C., & Hardy, M.C. (1929). "Later Development of Breast Fed and Artificially Fed Infants." *JAMA, 96,* 615-619.

153. Enlow, D.H., & Hans, M.G. (1996). "Essentials of Facial Growth." Philadelphia, PA: WB Saunders.

154. Yamada, T., Tanne, K., Miyamoto, K., & Yamauchi, K. (1997). "Influences of Nasal Respiratory Obstruction on Craniofacial Growth in Young Macaca Fuscata Monkeys." *Am J Orthod Dentofacial Orthop, 111*(1): 38-43.

155. Wright, J.L. (2001). "Diseases of the Small Airways." *Lung, 179*(6): 375-396.

156. Page, D.C., Sr. (2014). *Your Jaws – Your Life.* Baltimore: SmilePage Publishing, 33.

157. Vlahandonis, A., Walter, L.M., & Rosemary, R.S. (2013). "Does Treatment of SDB in Children Improve Cardiovascular Outcome?" *Sleep Med Rev, 17*(1): 75-85.

158. Guilleminault, C., & Huang, Y. S. (2017). "From Oral Facial Dysfunction to Dysmorphism and the Onset of Pediatric OSA." *Sleep Med Rev.*

159. Guilleminault, C., & Akhtar, F. (2015). "Pediatric Sleep-Disordered Breathing: New Evidence on its Development." *Sleep Med Rev, 24*, 46-56.

160. Huang, Y., & Guilleminault, C., (2013). "Pediatric Obstructive Sleep Apnea and the Critical Role of Oral-Facial Growth: Evidences." *Front Neurol, 3*(184): 1-7.

161. Marcus, C.L., Brooks, L.J., Ward, S.D., Draper, K.A., Gozal, D., Halbower, A.C., Jones, J., Lehmann, C., Schechter, M.S., Sheldon, S., Shiffman, R.N., & Spruyt, K. (2012). "Diagnosis and Management of Childhood Obstructive Sleep Apnea Syndrome." *Pediatrics, 130*(3): e714-e755.

162. Bonuck, K., Freeman, K., Chervin, R.D., & Xu, L. (2012). "Sleep-Disordered Breathing in a Population- Based Cohort: Behavioral Outcomes at 4 and 7 Years." *Pediatrics, 129*(4): 1-9.

163. Bonuck, K., Rao, T., & Xu, L. (2012, Oct.). "Pediatric Sleep Disorders and Special Educational Need at 8 Years: A Population-Based Cohort Study." *Pediatrics, 130*(4): 634-642.

164. Marangu, D., Jowi, C., Aswani, J., Wambani, S., & Nduati, R. (2014). "Prevalence and Associated Factors of Pulmonary Hypertension in Kenyan Children with Adenoid or Adenotonsillar Hypertrophy." *Int J Pediatr Otorhinolaryngol, 78*(8): 1381-1386.

165. Martha, V.F., da Silva Moreira, J., Martha, A.S., Velho, F.J., Eick, R.G., & Goncalves, S.C. (2013). "Reversal of Pulmonary Hypertension in Children After Adenoidectomy or Adenotonsillectomy." *Int J Pediatr Otorhinolaryngol, 77*(2): 237-240.

166. Ruoff, C.M., & Guilleminault, C. (2012, June). "Orthodontics and Sleep-Disordered Breathing." *Sleep breath, 16*(2): 271-273.

167. Camacho, M., Certal, V., Abdullatif, J., Zaghi, S., Ruoff, C.M., Capasso, R., & Kushida, C.A. (2015). "Myofunctional Therapy to Treat Obstructive Sleep Apnea: A Systematic Review and Meta-Analysis." *SLEEP, 38*(5): 669-675.

168. Ingram, D. (2018). *Sleep Apnea in Children: A Handbook for Families.* USA: Children's Mercy Hospital.

169. Gelb, M., & Hindin, H. (2016). *Gasp! Airway Health – The Hidden Path to Wellness.* USA: Gelb and Hindin.

170. Page, D.C., Sr. (2014). *Your Jaws – Your Life.* Baltimore: SmilePage Publishing.

171. Feig, C. (2011). "Exclusive Breastfeeding for Six Months Best for Babies Everywhere." Geneva, Switzerland: World Health Organization. Retrieved from http://www.who.int/mediacentre/news/statements/2011/breastfeeding_20110115/en/.

172. Kramer M.S., & Kakuma R. (2012). "Optimal Duration of Exclusive Breastfeeding." *Cochrane Database Syst Rev, 8*(8): (CD003517).

173. Widström, A.M., Lilja, G., Aaltomaa-Michalias, P., Dahllöf, A., Lintula, M., & Nissen, E. (2011). "Newborn Behaviour to Locate the Breast when Skin-to-Skin: A Possible Method for Enabling Early Self-Regulation." Acta Paediatr, 100(1): 79-85.

174. Girish, M., Mujawar, N., Gotmare, P., Paul, N., Punia, S., & Pandey, P. (2013). "Impact and Feasibility of Breast Crawl in a Tertiary Care Hospital." *J Perinatol, 33*(4): 288-291.

175. Heidarzadeh, M., Hakimi, S., Habibelahi, A., Mohammadi, M., & Shahrak, S.P. (2016). "Comparison of Breast Crawl Between Infants Delivered by Vaginal Delivery and Cesarean Section." *Breastfeed Med, 11*(6): 305-308.

176. McDonald, S.J., & Middleton, P. (2008). "Effect of Timing of Umbilical Cord Clamping of Term Infants on Maternal and Neonatal Outcomes." *Cochrane Database Syst Rev, 2*(2).

177. McDonald, S.J., & Middleton, P. (2008). "Effect of Timing of Umbilical Cord Clamping of Term Infants on Maternal and Neonatal Outcomes." *Cochrane Database Syst Rev, 2*(2).

178. Speer, C.P., Schatz, R., & Gahr, M. (1985). "Function of Breast Milk Macrophages." *Monatsschrift Kinderheilkunde: Organ der Deutschen Gesellschaft fur Kinderheilkunde, 133*(11): 913-917.

179. Cummings, N.P., Neifert, M.R., Pabst, M.J., & Johnston, R.B. (1985). "Oxidative Metabolic Response and Microbicidal Activity of Human Milk Macrophages: Effect of Lipopolysaccharide and Muramyl Dipeptide." *Infect and Immun, 49*(2): 435-439.

180. Queiroz, V.A.D.O., Assis, A.M.O., Júnior, R., & da Costa, H. (2013). "Protective Effect of Human Lactoferrin in the Gastrointestinal Tract." *Revista Paulista de Pediatria, 31*(1): 90-95.

181. Genna, C.W. (2017). *Supporting Sucking Skills in Breastfeeding Infants.* Woodhaven, NY: Jones and Bartlett Learning.

182. Walker, M. (2016). "Nipple Shields: What We Know, What We Wish We Knew, and How Best to Use Them." *Clinical Lactation, 7*(3): 100-107.

183. Boyd, K.L. (2012). "Darwinian Dentistry Part 2: Early Childhood Nutrition, Dentofacial Development, and Chronic Disease." *JAOS.* 28-32.

184. Boyd, K.L. (2011). "Darwinian Dentistry Part 1: An Evolutionary Perspective on the Etiology of Malocclusion." *JAOS,* 34-40.

185. Lin, S. (2018). *The Dental Diet: The Surprising Link Between Your Teeth, Real Food, and Life-Changing Natural Health.* USA, Australia, UK, Canada, India: Hay House, Inc.

186. Cockley, L., & Lehman, A. (2015, Winter). "The Ortho Missing Link: Could it be Tied to the Tongue?" *Journal of the American Orthodontic Society,* 18-21.

187. Hazelbaker, A.K. (2010). *Tongue-Tie: Morphogenesis, Impact, Assessment, and Treatment.* Columbus, OH: Aiden and Eva Press.

188. Genna, C.W. (2017). "The Influence of Anatomic and Structural Issues on Sucking Skills." In C.W. Genna (Ed.), *Supporting Sucking Skills in Breastfeeding Infants* (3rd ed., pp. 209-267). Woodhaven, NY: Jones and Bartlett Learning.

189. Martinelli, R.L., Marchesan, I.Q., Gusmão, R.J., Rodrigues, A., & Berretin-Felix, G. (2014). "Histological Characteristics of Altered Human Lingual Frenulum." *Int J Pediatr Child Health, 2,* 6-9.

190. Acevedo, A.C., da Fonseca, J.A.C., Grinham, J., Doudney, K., Gomes, R.R., de Paula, L.M., & Stanier, P. (2010). "Autosomal-Dominant Ankyloglossia and Tooth Number Anomalies." *J Dent Res, 89*(2): 128-132.

191. Han, S.H., Kim, M.C., Choi, Y.S., Lim, J.S., & Han, K.T. (2012). "A Study on the Genetic Inheritance of Ankyloglossia Based on Pedigree Analysis." *Arch Plast Surg, 39*(4): 329-332.

192. Klockars, T., & Pitkäranta, A. (2009b). "Inheritance of Ankyloglossia (Tongue-Tie)." *Clin Genet, 75*(1): 98- 99.

193. Coryllos, E., Genna, C.W., & Salloum, A.C. (2004). "Congenital Tongue-Tie and its Impact on Breastfeeding." *Breastfeeding: Best for Mother and Baby,* 1-6.

194. Cheng, M.C., Enlow, D.H., Papsidero, M., Broadbent Jr, B.H., Oyen, O., & Sabat, M. (1988). "Developmental Effects of Impaired Breathing in the Face of the Growing Child." *Angle Orthod, 58*(4): 309- 320.

195. Guilleminault, C., & Huang, Y.S. (2017). "From Oral Facial Dysfunction to Dysmorphism and the Onset of Pediatric OSA." *Sleep Med Rev.*

196. Lundberg, J.O.N., & Weitzberg, E. (1999). "Nasal Nitric Oxide in Man." *Thorax, 54*(10): 947-952.

197. Marangu, D., Jowi, C., Aswani, J., Wambani, S., & Nduati, R. (2014). "Prevalence and Associated Factors of Pulmonary Hypertension in Kenyan Children with Adenoid or Adenotonsillar Hypertrophy." *Int J Pediatr Otorhinolaryngol, 78*(8): 1381-1386.

198. Schlenker, W.L., Jennings, B.D., Jeiroudi, M.T., & Caruso, J.M. (2000). "The Effects of Chronic Absence of Active Nasal Respiration on the Growth of the Skull: A Pilot Study." *Am J Orthod Dentofacial Orthop, 117*(6): 706-713.

199. Francis, D.O., Chinnadurai, S., Morad, A., Epstein, R.A., Kohanim, S., Krishnaswami, S., Sathe. N.A., & McPheeters, M.L. (2015, May). "Treatments for Ankyloglossia and Ankyloglossia with Concomitant Lip-Tie." Comparative Effectiveness Review No. 149. (Prepared by the Vanderbilt Evidence-Based Practice Center under Contract No. 290-2012-00009-I.) AHRQ Publication No. 15-EHC011-EF. Rockville, MD: Agency for Healthcare Research and Quality. Retrieved from http://www.effectivehealthcare.ahrq.gov/search-for-guides-reviews-and-reports/?pageaction=displayproduct&productid=2073.

200. Convissar, R.A., Hazelbaker, A., Kaplan, M.A., & Vitruk, P. (2017). *Color Atlas of Infant Tongue-Tie and Lip-Tie Laser Frenectomy.* Columbus, OH: PanSophia Press, LLC.

201. Boshart, C. (2015). *Demystify the Tongue Tie: Methods to Confidently Analyze and Treat a Tethered Tongue.* Ellijay, GA: Speech Dynamics.

202. Merkel-Walsh, R. & Overland, L.L. (in press). *Functional Assessment and Remediation of Tethered Oral Tissues.* Charleston, SC: TalkTools.

203. Pine, P. (2018). *Please Release Me: The Tethered Oral Tissue (TOT) Puzzle.* USA: Minibuk.

204. Kotlow, L.A. (2016). *SOS 4 TOTS: Tethered Oral Tissues, Tongue-Ties & Lip Ties.* New York: Troy Bookmakers.

205. Genna, C.W. (2017). *Supporting Sucking Skills in Breastfeeding Infants.* Woodhaven, NY: Jones and Bartlett Learning.

206. Horsfall, C. (2013). *Tongue Tie: Breastfeeding and Beyond. A Parents' Guide to Diagnosis, Division and Aftercare.* Kindle Direct Publishing.

207. Fernando, C. (1998). *Tongue Tie - From Confusion to Clarity: A Guide to the Diagnosis and Treatment of Ankyloglossia.* Australia: Tandem Publications.

208. Hazelbaker, A.K. (2010). *Tongue-Tie: Morphogenesis, Impact, Assessment, and Treatment.* Columbus, OH: Aiden and Eva Press.

209. Colson, S.D., Meek, J.H., & Hawdon, J.M. (2008). "Optimal Positions for the Release of Primitive Neonatal Reflexes Stimulating Breastfeeding." *Early Hum Dev, 84*, 441-449.

210. Colson, S. (2005). "Maternal Breastfeeding Positions: Have We Got It Right?" (1). *Pract Midwife, 8*(10): 24, 26-27.

211. Colson, S. (2005). "Maternal Breastfeeding Positions: Have We Got It Right?" (1). *Pract Midwife, 8*(11): 29-32.

212. Bagdade, J.D., & Hirsch, J. (1966). "Gestational and Dietary Influences on the Lipid Content of the Infant Buccal Fat Pad." *Proc Soc Exp Biol Med, 122*(2): 616-619.

213. Einarsson-Backes, L.M., Deitz, J., Price, R., Glass, R., & Hays, R. (1994). "The Effect of Oral Support on Sucking Efficiency in Preterm Infants." *Am J Occup Ther, 48*(6): 490-498.

214. Hill, A.S. (2005). "The Effects of Nonnutritive Sucking and Oral Support on the Feeding Efficiency of Preterm Infants." *Newborn Infant Nurs Rev, 5*(3): 133-141.

215. Hill, A.S., Kurkowski, T.B., & Garcia, J. (2000). "Oral Support Measures Used in Feeding the Preterm Infant." *Nursing Research, 49*(1): 2-10.

216. Jackson, I.T. (1999). "Anatomy of the Buccal Fat Pad and its Clinical Significance." *Plast Reconstr Surg, 103*(7): 2061-2063.

217. Patil, R., Singh, S., & Subba Reddy, V.V. (2003, Dec.). "Herniation of the Buccal Fat Pad into the Oral Cavity: A Case Report." *J Indian Sot Pedo Prev Dent, 21*(4).

218. Ponrartana, S., Patil, S., Aggabao, P.C., Pavlova, Z., Devaskar, S.U., & Gilsanz, V. (2014). "Brown Adipose Tissue in the Buccal Fat Pad During Infancy." *PloS one, 9*(2): e89533.

219. Racz, L., Maros, T.N., & Seres-Sturm, L. (1989). "Structural Characteristics and Functional Significance of the Buccal Fat Pad (Corpus Adiposum Buccae)." *Morphol Embryol, 35*(2): 73-77.

220. Tostevin, P.M.J., & Ellis, H. (1995). "The Buccal Pad of Fat: A Review." *Clin Anat, 8*(6): 403-406.

221. Speer C.P., Schatz R., & Gahr M. (1985). "Function of Breast Milk Macrophages." *Monatsschr Kinderheilkd, 133*(11): 913-917.

222. Cummings, N.P., Neifert, M.R., Pabst, M.J., & Johnston, R.B. (1985). "Oxidative Metabolic Response and Microbicidal Activity of Human Milk Macrophages: Effect of Lipopolysaccharide and Muramyl Dipeptide." *Infect Immun, 49*(2): 435-439.

223. Speer, C.P., Schatz, R., & Gahr, M. (1985). "Function of Breast Milk Macrophages." *Monatsschrift Kinderheilkunde: Organ der Deutschen Gesellschaft fur Kinderheilkunde, 133*(11): 913-917.

224. Cummings, N.P., Neifert, M.R., Pabst, M.J., & Johnston, R.B. (1985). "Oxidative Metabolic Response and Microbicidal Activity of Human Milk Macrophages: Effect of Lipopolysaccharide and Muramyl Dipeptide." *Infection and Immunity, 49*(2): 435-439.

225. Queiroz, V.A.D.O., Assis, A.M.O., Júnior, R., & da Costa, H. (2013). "Protective Effect of Human Lactoferrin in the Gastrointestinal Tract." *Revista Paulista de Pediatria, 31*(1): 90-95.

226. West, D., & Marasco, L. (2009). *The Breastfeeding Mother's Guide to Making More Milk*. Columbus, OH: McGraw Hill.

227. West. D, & Marasco, L (2009). *The Breastfeeding Mother's Guide to Making More Milk*. Columbus, OH: McGraw Hill.

228. Zemlin, W.R. (1998). *Speech and Hearing Science: Anatomy and Physiology* (4th ed.). Boston: Allyn and Bacon, 547.

229. Ginsberg, I.A., & White, T.P. (1978). "Otological Considerations in Audiology." In J. Katz (Ed.), *Handbook of Clinical Audiology* (2nd ed., pp. 8-22), Baltimore, MD: Williams & Wilkins, 13.

230. Goetzinger, C.P. (1978). "Word Discrimination Testing." In J. Katz (Ed.), *Handbook of Clinical Audiology* (2nd ed., pp. 149-158), Baltimore, MD: Williams & Wilkins, 151.

231. Sachs, J. "The Emergence of Intentional Communication." In J.B. Gleason (Ed.), *The Development of Language* (3rd ed., pp. 39-64). New York: Macmillan Publishing Company, 40.

232. Geddes, D.T., Kent, J.C., Mitoulas, L.R., & Hartmann, P.E. (2008). "Tongue Movement and Intra-Oral Vacuum in Breastfeeding Infants." *Early Hum Dev, 84*(7): 471-477.

233. Elad, D., Kozlovsky, P., Blum, O., Laine, A.F., Ming, J.P., Botzer, E., Dollberg, S., Zelicovich, M., & Sira, L.B. (2014, Apr). "Biomechanics of Milk Extraction During Breast-Feeding." *Proceedings of the National Academy of Sciences for the United Stated of America, 111*(14): 5230-5235.

234. Genna, C.W. (2017). *Supporting Sucking Skills in Breastfeeding Infants* (3rd ed.). Woodhaven, NY: Jones and Bartlett Learning.

235. Genna, C.W., (2017). "The Influence of Anatomic and Structural Issues on Sucking Skills." In C.W. Genna (Ed.), *Supporting Sucking Skills in Breastfeeding Infants* (3rd ed., pp. 209-267). Woodhaven, NY: Jones and Bartlett Learning.

236. Genna, C.W., & Sandora, L. (2017). "Breastfeeding: Normal Sucking and Swallowing." In C.W. Genna (Ed.), *Supporting Sucking Skills in Breastfeeding Infants* (3rd ed., pp. 1-48). Woodhaven, NY: Jones and Bartlett Learning.

237. Guilleminault, C., & Huang, Y. (2017). "From Oral Facial Dysfunction and Onset of Pediatric OSA: Evidences." *Sleep Med Rev.*

238. Guilleminault, C., & Huang, Y. (2017). "From Oral Facial Dysfunction and Onset of Pediatric OSA: Evidences." *Sleep Med Rev.*

239. Santos-Neto, E.T., Oliveira, A.E., Barbosa, R.W., Zandonade, E., & Oliveira, L. (2012). "The Influence of Sucking Habits on Occlusion Development in the First 36 Months." *Dental Press J Orthod, 17*(4): 96-104.

240. Merrill, P. (2008). *Feedback from Lactation Consultant* – Baltimore, MD: http://www.nurturingnaturallylc.net/.

241. Satter, E. (2000). *Child of Mine: Feeding with Love and Good Sense.* Boulder, CO: Bull Publishing Company, 162.

242. Satter, E. (2000). *Child of Mine: Feeding with Love and Good Sense.* Boulder, CO: Bull Publishing Company, 165-166, 206-207.

243. Satter, E. (2000). *Child of Mine: Feeding with Love and Good Sense.* Boulder, CO: Bull Publishing Company, 218.

244. Satter, E. (2000). *Child of Mine: Feeding with Love and Good Sense.* Boulder, CO: Bull Publishing Company, 231.

245. Northrup, C. (2005). *Mother-Daughter Wisdom: Creating a Legacy of Physical and Emotional Health.* New York: Bantam Dell, 212-214.

246. Batmanghelidj, F. (1997). *Your Body's Many Cries for Water.* Vienna, VA: Global Health Solutions, 8.

247. Batmanghelidj, F. (1997). *Your Body's Many Cries for Water.* Vienna, VA: Global Health Solutions, 13.

248. Batmanghelidj, F. (1997). *Your Body's Many Cries for Water.* Vienna, VA: Global Health Solutions.

249. Satter, E. (2000). *Child of Mine: Feeding with Love and Good Sense.* Boulder, CO: Bull Publishing Company, 176-177.

250. Satter, E. (2000). *Child of Mine: Feeding with Love and Good Sense.* Boulder, CO: Bull Publishing Company, 509.

251. Karp, H. (2002). *The Happiest Baby on the Block*. New York: Bantam Dell, 4.

252. Rosenfeld-Johnson, S. (1999). *A Three-Part Treatment Plan for Oral-Motor Therapy*. Baltimore, MD: Innovative Therapists International, Workshop.

253. Yilmaz, G., Caylan, N., Karacan, C.D., Bodur, I., & Gokcay, G. (2014). "Effect of Cup Feeding and Bottle Feeding on Breastfeeding in Late Preterm Infants: A Randomized Controlled Study." *J Hum Lact, 30*(2): 174-179.

254. Gomes, C.F., Trezza, E., Murade, E., & Padovani, C.R. (2006). "Surface Electromyography of Facial Muscles During Natural and Artificial Feeding of Infants." *Jornal de Pediatria, 82*(2): 103-109.

255. Abouelfettoh, A.M., Dowling, D.A., Dabash, S.A., Elguindy, S.R., & Seoud, I.A. (2008). "Cup Versus Bottle Feeding for Hospitalized Late Preterm Infants in Egypt: A Quasi-Experimental Study." *Int Breastfeed J*, 3(1): 27.

256. Gupta, A., Khanna, K., & Chattree, S. (1999). "Brief Report. Cup Feeding: An Alternative to Bottle Feeding in a Neonatal Intensive Care Unit." *J Tropical Pediatr, 45*(2): 108-110.

257. Marinelli, K.A., Burke, G.S., & Dodd, V.L. (2001). "A Comparison of the Safety of Cupfeedings and Bottlefeedings in Premature Infants Whose Mothers Intend to Breastfeed." *J Perinatol, 21*(6): 350.

258. Tinanoff, N., & Palmer, C.A. (2000). "Dietary Determinants of Dental Caries and Dietary Recommendations for Preschool Children." *Journal Public Health Dent, 60*(3): 197-206.

259. Potock, M. (n.d.). "Why You May Want to Skip the Sippy Cup for Your Baby." *Parents*. Retrieved from https://www.parents.com/baby/feeding/center/why-you-may-want-to-skip-the-sippy-cup-for-your-baby/.

260. Potock, M. (2014, Jan). "Step Away from the Sippy Cup!" *The ASHA Leader Blog*. Retrieved from https://blog.asha.org/2014/01/09/step-away-from-the-sippy-cup/.

261. Potock, M. (2017, Feb). "Sippy Cups: 3 Reasons to Skip Them and What to Offer Instead." *The ASHA Leader Blog*. Retrieved from https://blog.asha.org/2017/02/28/sippy-cups-3-reasons-to-skip-them-and-what-to-offer-instead/.

262. Rosenfeld-Johnson, S. (1999). *A Three-Part Treatment Plan for Oral-Motor Therapy*. (Baltimore: Innovative Therapists International). Workshop.

263. Bahr, D. (2010). *Nobody Ever Told Me (or My Mother) That! Everything from Bottles and Breathing to Healthy Speech Development*. Arlington, TX: Sensory World/Future Horizons.

264. Lowsky, D.C. (2011). *Tips & Techniques Exercise Book for the Grabber Family*. Lugoff, SC: ARK Therapeutic Services.

265. Oetter, P., Richter, E.W., & Frick, S.M. (1995). *M.O.R.E.: Integrating the Mouth with Sensory and Postural Functions* (2nd ed.). Hugo, MN: PDP Press, Inc.

266. Johnson, S. R. (2009). *OPT (Oral Placement Therapy) for Speech Clarity and Feeding.* Charleston, SC: TalkTools.

267. Field, T. (2000). *Touch Therapy.* New York: Churchill Livingstone.

268. Potock, M. (2018). *Adventures in Veggieland: Help Your Kids Learn to Love Vegetables with 100 Easy Activities and Recipes.* New York, NY: The Experiment.

269. Ripton, N., & Potock, M. (2016). *Baby Self-Feeding: Solid Food Solutions to Create Lifelong, Healthy Eating Habits.* Beverly, MA: Quarto Publishing Group.

270. Satter, E. (2000). *Child of Mine: Feeding with Love and Good Sense.* Boulder, CO: Bull Publishing Company.

271. Potock, M. (2010). *Happy Mealtimes with Happy Kids: How to Teach Your Child About the Joy of Food.* Longmont, Colorado: My Munch Bug.

272. Rowell, K., & McGlothlin, J. (2015). *Helping Your Child with Extreme Picky Eating: A Step-by-Step Guide for Overcoming Selective Eating, Food Aversion, and Feeding Disorders.* Oakland, CA: New Harbinger Publications.

273. Satter, E. (1987). *How to Get Your Kid to Eat … but Not Too Much.* Palo Alto, CA: Bull Publishing Company.

274. Ernsperger, L., & Stegen-Hanson, T. (2004). *Just Take a Bite: Easy, Effective Answers to Food Aversions and Eating Challenges.* Arlington, TX: Future Horizons, Inc.

275. Fernando, N., & Potock, M. (2015). *Raising a Healthy, Happy Eater: A Stage-by-Stage Guide to Setting Your Child on the Path to Adventurous Eating.* New York, NY: The Experiment.

Author Bio

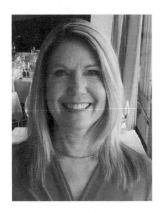

Diane Bahr is a visionary with a mission. For almost forty years, she has treated children and adults with feeding, motor speech, and mouth function problems. While she is a speech-language pathologist by training, she has also honed her skills as a feeding therapist, published author, international speaker, university instructor, and business owner. Diane co-owns Ages and Stages®, LLC with her husband and business manager Joe Bahr. She is also a mother and a grandmother.

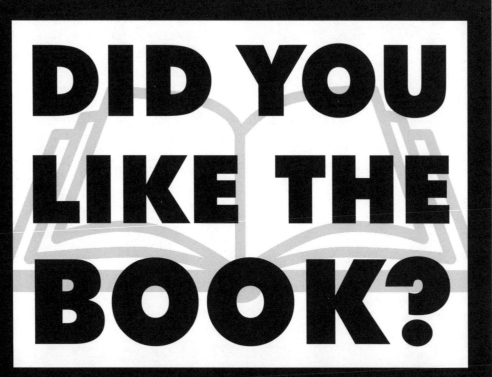

DID YOU LIKE THE BOOK?

Rate it and share your opinion.

amazon.com   BARNES&NOBLE
BOOKSELLERS
www.bn.com

Not what you expected? Tell us!

Most negative reviews occur when the book did not reach expectation. Did the description build any expectations that were not met? Let us know how we can do better.

Please drop us a line at *info@fhautism.com.*

Thank you so much for your support!

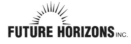

FUTURE HORIZONS INC.